THE
FOOT
BOOK

Ralph,

Thank you for being my patient.

The Foot Book Doctor

THE FOOT BOOK
Fast Foot Facts from the Foot Care Front Lines
Copyright © 2023 Dr. Paul Betschart

ISBN: 978-1-956220-29-2

Expert Press
2 Shepard Hills Court
Little Rock, AR 72223
www.ExpertPress.net

Editing by Heidi Ward
Proofreading by Geeha Barret-Fernandez
Text design and composition by Emily Fritz
Cover design by Casey Fritz

THE

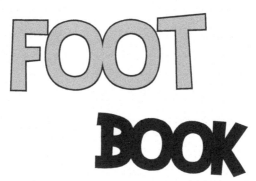

FOOT

BOOK

FAST FOOT FACTS
FROM THE FOOT CARE FRONT LINES

DR. PAUL BETSCHART
THE FOOT BOOK DOCTOR

Contents

PREFACE

In my more than twenty-seven years of practice as a foot and ankle specialist, I have had the privilege of helping thousands of people attain better health from the ground up. This book is dedicated to everyone who puts their feet in my hands. It is my hope that this book can help others achieve better foot and ankle health, which can then support healthy activities and the ability to work in jobs that require standing, walking, or climbing. This book is not designed to be a medical reference text. It is a compendium of the knowledge and experience I have gained from over a quarter century of foot and ankle care. It focuses on the most common conditions that I see on a regular basis as a practitioner. Where possible, I keep the medical jargon to a minimum to make the text understandable to the general public. I hope you find this information valuable. I welcome any and all questions and comments from readers. I can be reached at info@danburypodiatrist.com.

ONE

Heel Pain and Plantar Fasciitis

BACKGROUND INFORMATION

By far, the most common cause of heel pain is a condition called plantar fasciitis. This condition is an injury to a ligament on the bottom of the foot called the plantar fascia. It runs the length of the foot, from the heel bone to the base of the toes. The most common part of the plantar fascia to be injured is under the heel where it attaches to the heel bone. The body responds to this injury with inflammation, which is perceived as pain. This ligament is one of the most important stabilizing structures of the arch of the foot. A common cause of injury to the plantar fascia is the lack of arch support in shoes. Other causes include direct trauma, such as stepping on a hard object; overuse, like building up running mileage too fast; and inflammatory conditions, such as rheumatoid arthritis. Less common causes of heel pain include fractures of the heel bone, bone tumors, bone cysts, foreign bodies, skin tumors, and soft-tissue or bone infections. These causes of heel pain would need to be diagnosed and treated by a medical professional. This chapter will focus on managing the most common cause of heel pain—plantar fasciitis.

REST

Pain after an injury is the body's signal to us to rest that part. Rest is the first part in the healing process. Rest doesn't necessarily mean you can't put weight on your foot or that you must stick to bed rest. Relative rest is usually sufficient and just means reducing your level of activity below that which causes pain to increase. For example, if running causes pain to increase, stopping running and only walking would provide the relative rest needed. Sometimes, a reduction in mileage or intensity will be sufficient. Occasionally, it may be necessary to off-load, or limit pressure on, the area with a walking boot or to use crutches or a knee scooter for completely non-weight-bearing mobility.

Reducing inflammation is also important in this phase. Cold application is a great way to reduce inflammation. Twenty minutes on, twenty minutes off around the clock for the first forty-eight hours is ideal, but if that is not possible, doing so for as much of the day as possible will help. An easy way to apply cold at work is to freeze a plastic water bottle and rest your foot on it, gently rolling the arch on the bottle. Gel packs, crushed ice, or frozen peas are other alternatives for applying cold. Anti-inflammatory medications such as aspirin, ibuprofen, naproxen, etc. can be taken for five to seven days to reduce inflammation. CBD products are an alternative way to reduce inflammation and pain naturally. Topical pain creams can help with symptom control, but they do not have anti-inflammatory properties. For example, arnica is a homeopathic anti-inflammatory topical remedy that can be effective for pain relief. Protecting the heel area is very important during this phase. Heel cups made out of silicone or rubber can be used for protection while walking. Avoid flat shoes or sandals, as they increase the heel strike force. Elevating the heel slightly also takes tension off the plantar fascia and supinates (or raises the arch of) the foot, which provides stability. A standard running shoe should have the right amount of heel lift. Dress shoes and boots should be limited to shorter than two inches of heel. Night splints are a good way to protect the foot when sleeping or resting. These can be found online or through a medical professional. Elastic arch bandages and compression socks are also helpful in resting the plantar fascia. One to two weeks of using these recovery methods should help reduce symptoms enough to begin the rehabilitation phase.

REHABILITATION

The rehabilitation phase is divided into three components: support, stretch, and strength.

SUPPORT

To allow the plantar fascia to heal properly, tension or strain on the tissue must be reduced. To accomplish this, we must support the arch of the foot. Since the plantar fascia runs the length of the bottom of the foot, supporting the center of the arch will relieve strain on the insertion point of the ligament on the heel bone, where the injury usually occurs. There are several effective support strategies available.

Taping:

Various taping techniques and materials are available to provide support to the plantar fascia. A simple and effective taping technique is called the Campbell's rest strap. This technique uses quarter-inch athletic tape in short strips. Starting just forward of the heel pad, place a strip across the bottom of the foot, starting on the outside below the ankle bone and ending on the inside of the foot below the ankle bone. Add more strips in the same manner, overlapping each other by half of the strip. End when you reach the ball of the foot. Anchoring strips can be used over the ends of the strips on the sides of the foot. The tape can be left in place as long as it is providing support. The length of time it is effective will vary based on activity level, sweating, water exposure, etc. You can have a buddy apply this for you if flexibility issues prevent reaching the bottom of the foot.

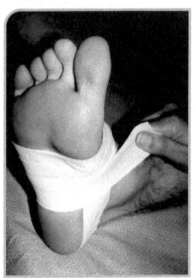

There are a variety of elastic supports commercially available that range from compression socks to arch binders to elastic with rubber arch supports. Though less effective than taping, these have the advantage of being removable and reusable.

Insoles:

Insoles have the advantages of convenience, comfort, and durability. However, the majority of insoles found in stores provide only cushioning and little, if any, arch support. Insoles with firm plastic arch forms are the most effective type of over-the-counter (OTC) insole. Some brands with these are Superfeet®, PowerSteps®, and Sorbothane®. These can usually be found at sporting goods stores, running stores, or online. These types fit the average foot well. People with extremes in their arch height—low or high—may not be comfortable in OTC devices and may need to have theirs custom-made. Insoles have the advantages of convenience, comfort, and durability. When using insoles, I recommend that the foot be supported for at least six months to allow the tissue to fully heal and remodel.

STRETCH

Stretching exercises and self-massages help release tension on the involved soft tissues, improve blood flow, and realign tissue fibers. Stretching also addresses some of the underlying biomechanical imbalances that contributed to the injury.

The most important area to stretch for most foot and ankle conditions is the Achilles tendon/calf muscle complex. This tendon attaches to the back of the heel bone, and its fibers extend to the bottom of the foot and blend with the plantar fascia fibers. Stretching this tendon will reduce tension on the plantar fascia.

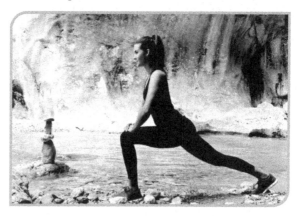

The easiest stretch to accomplish this is the wall push up, or sprinter's stretch. Stand a few feet from a wall with feet together and toes pointed toward the wall. Place both hands on the wall and lean forward, bending at the ankle and keeping your body as straight as possible. When you feel a comfortable stretch in the tendon or calf muscle, hold the stretch for ten seconds, then relax for several seconds. Repeat the ten-second stretches ten times. As your mobility improves, you can hold the stretch for up to thirty seconds to improve flexibility. Keep your knee fully extended in the initial set. Next, repeat the ten-second stretches with a slight bend in the knees. Do ten repetitions. This will stretch another part of the calf muscle, the soleus. Some people find it easier to stretch one leg at a time in a lunge position. An alternative to this stretch is the towel stretch. Wrap a towel or an exercise band under the ball of the foot and pull the foot up toward the leg. Hold for ten seconds, and repeat the holds ten times as before.

To stretch the plantar fascia, sit on the edge of a bed or chair with your foot flat on the floor. Lift your heel and roll up on your toes. You will feel the stretch in the bottom of the foot. Hold for ten seconds for ten repetitions. While the plantar fascia is not a ligament, it does function as one and doesn't stretch as much, so don't force it. Be careful with this stretch if you have arthritic toe joints. This stretch can be performed first thing in the morning when getting out of bed to help with the first step pain that is common with plantar fasciitis.

Self-massages of the plantar fascia should be performed for ten to fifteen minutes daily. A firm ball or a foam roller works best. A plastic water bottle or aluminum can can be used as an alternative. Position the ball in the center of the arch of the foot. Roll the foot from back to front, using as much pressure as is comfortable. Avoid rolling directly over the heel, where the plantar fascia attaches. Another area to massage is the calf muscle fascia. This area is on the back of the leg just below the thick portion of the calf muscle. While seated on the floor or couch, rest your leg on the ball or roller and roll from the calf muscle to where the Achilles tendon starts, about four inches above the heel bone.

For a more effective stretch or massage, warm up the soft tissue prior to starting. Soaking in a solution of Epsom salt and warm water works well. Mix one cup of Epsom salt per gallon of warm water. Make sure the water is not too hot by using a thermometer. The temperature should be no higher than 120 degrees F. Soak for ten to fifteen minutes. Foot soaking devices are available that agitate the water and keep it warm, but simply using a deep basin works fine.

Alternative heating modalities include gel packs, electric heating pads, and infrared devices.

STRENGTH

Once pain has subsided and mobility has improved, the final phase of rehabilitation can begin. The small muscles of the foot are difficult to isolate in order to exercise, but it is worth the effort since these muscles help stabilize the foot during walking.

Towel curls are an easy exercise to start with. Place the foot on a towel and try to scrunch up the towel with your toes. Do this for five to ten minutes. When you get good at the towel curl, you can try picking up a pencil or even marbles with your toes. One of the most effective exercises for the arch-stabilizing muscles is a yoga technique called Short Foot. It can be difficult to master, but the resulting improvement in stability and balance is unmatched by other exercises. Searching this technique on YouTube will bring up several instructional videos. As with most yoga techniques, there are many interpretations of the form and focus. My colleague Emily Splichal, DPM, has several videos on her website (www.barefootstrong.com) that explain and demonstrate it well.

RECURRENCE PREVENTION

Once symptoms have been resolved, the main objective is to keep the problem from coming back. The first step is to try to identify any causative factors that may have brought about the injury, such as training errors, inappropriate footwear, direct trauma, etc., and take steps to avoid that issue in the future. If you cannot identify a cause, the injury is likely the result of a biomechanical imbalance of the foot or leg. This is when you will likely need to seek the advice of a foot and ankle specialist. Look for a specialist certified by the American Board of Foot and Ankle Surgery or the American Board of Foot and Ankle Medicine.

Even after symptoms have stopped, maintain your stretching program. Focus on stretching the Achilles tendon daily and after sporting activities. This tendon tends to get tight easily, especially in athletes and those who wear high heels. Regular stretching can help prevent this and many other foot injuries.

You should continue to use a firm, supportive insole for at least six months. If a biomechanical cause is suspected, support should be maintained for the future. If symptoms return despite the use of a good OTC arch support, you may need a custom foot orthotic. Again, this is where consultation with a foot and ankle specialist would be appropriate.

TWO

Nail Conditions

NAIL FUNGUS

Nail fungus, or onychomycosis, is one of the most common conditions we treat in podiatry offices. Fungal infections of the nail unit can result in changes of the appearance and quality of the nail plate. The nails often become discolored, thick, and brittle. Keratotic debris, which is made up of dead skin cells and fungal organisms, can form between the nail plate and the nail bed (the specialized skin beneath the nail.) Fungal infections usually begin with a break in the nail's natural barriers to infection, usually through trauma such as stubbing the toe or cutting the nails too short. The fungal organisms gain access to under the surface of the nail and start to grow, using the nail plate as food. Keratotic debris that forms can lift the nail plate up further, allowing the fungal organisms to spread to more of the nail. If the infection reaches the nail root, nail growth is disrupted, resulting in thickening and irregularity of the nail plate. The fact that the infection is largely under the nail plate makes treating this condition difficult with topical agents alone. A variant of fungal nail infections, white superficial onychomycosis, occurs on the top surface of the nail, making it easier to treat with topical medications.

A dermatophyte, which means "skin lover," is the most common class of fungi that causes nail infections. It is in same class of fungi that causes skin fungal infections such as athlete's foot and ringworm. Other, less common organisms that cause nail infections are saprophytes and yeasts. It is important to diagnose the infecting organisms in order to guide treatment decisions. The most accurate testing available today uses genetic sequencing to screen for many different organisms. These tests are sensitive and only require small sample amounts. Current testing can identify bacterial involvement as well. Microscopic evaluation can confirm the presence of fungal organisms and rule out other causes of nail dystrophy.

Treating nail fungal infections is usually multimodal. The first step is to reduce nail thickness by cutting and/or filing the nail down, which is called debridement. This can help reduce fungal load, enhance topical agent penetration, help reduce symptoms, and improve nail appearance. Topical antifungals such as tolnaftate 1 percent solution should be applied to the nails one to two times daily. Penetrating agents such as urea can help improve topical antifungals' effectiveness. However, most moderate-to-severe infections usually need oral antifungal therapy.

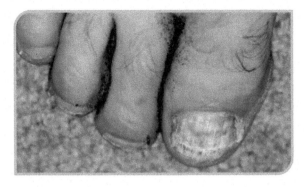

Modern oral agents are safe for most patients, but patients with active liver disease should be monitored closely by their internist during oral antifungal therapy. Employing a pulsed, or interrupted, dosing regimen can improve safety. Agents are typically taken for one week at a time with pulses repeated between one and three months apart. Effectiveness of pulse dosing has been shown to be similar to continuous dosing. The length of pulsed treatment varies based on nail growth speed and is typically six to twelve months, whereas continuous dosing is usually ninety days for toenail fungal conditions. Liver function testing would be needed monthly when using continuous dosing. After the three months of continuous dosing, the nail will be observed for an additional three to six months to make sure the nail continues to grow out and clear the remainder of the nail. The new nail grows to replace the infected nail, which is trimmed off the end as growth continues. It is important to continue treatment until the new nail completely grows in. Recurrence is uncommon after complete clearance; however, some people have a higher susceptibility to fungal infections and may need closer observation and to use preventive measures.

The most common adverse effect that concerns most people using oral antifungals is the potential for liver toxicity. As noted above, this is exceedingly rare for modern antifungals, but anyone with current or suspected liver disease should be considered for liver function testing prior to starting oral antifungals. It is not necessary to monitor liver function tests during treatment if using pulse dosing due to the reduced amount of medication and the interval between pulses. If patients experience jaundice, unexplained abdominal pain, or white-colored stools while taking oral antifungals, they should repeat a liver function test.

Oral antifungal selection should be based on testing of the nails, if possible. The most commonly used oral antifungal for nail infections is terbinafine. Other effective agents are itraconazole and fluconazole.

For patients who cannot or will not take oral antifungals, other methods can be employed to attack the fungus under the nail plate, such as laser therapy. Laser devices of various wavelengths and powers have been employed for nail fungus. I have found that photodynamic therapy (PTD) using exposure to low-level laser energy after applying a photosensitizing dye, such as methylene blue, to be highly effective at treating nail fungal and bacterial infections. PDT regimens are typically performed every two weeks for two to four months

Some patients have repeatedly negative fungal cultures but may have bacteria isolated from their samples. It is unclear at this time whether this bacterial isolation represents a genuine clinical infection or a contamination.

More research needs to be done on this subject to provide a clearer answer. I have had success treating patients with fungal negative, bacterial positive nails using topical antibiotic compounds based on the results of genetic sequencing and resistant-gene identification. Treatment with these agents is typically needed for six to twelve months based on the rate of nail growth.

INGROWN TOENAILS

Ingrown toenails are a painful condition that can affect people of all ages. They are commonly caused by improper nail trimming, trauma to the toes, ill-fitting footwear, fungal infections of the nail, and genetic nail deformities. The usual signs of ingrown nails are pain, swelling, and redness of the soft tissues around the nail. Drainage of clear to cloudy fluid from around the nail may be seen. Self-treatment is usually ineffective, and delaying treatment can risk spreading infection, infecting the bone, and even leading to amputation. Risks are greater in people who have compromised immune systems or who have poor circulation. Medical personnel commonly prescribe topical and oral antibiotics; however, antibiotics alone are rarely curative. Often, the embedded nail fragment acts as a foreign body, causing continued pain and swelling even after the infection is treated. Recurrence of the infection is typical without definitive treatment. Partial nail removal along with drainage of any infection is usually an effective cure. This short procedure can be easily and safely performed in an office under local anesthetic. Afterward, the patient or caregiver will need to perform simple wound care to the area daily for one to two weeks using topical antibiotic compounds. Oral antibiotic agents are rarely needed unless the infection has spread beyond the nail area. The nail will return to normal shape within six months.

In patients with repeated ingrown nails, permanent removal of the offending portion of the nail may be necessary to prevent recurrence. The most common type of permanent partial nail removal is chemical matrixectomy. This procedure combines a partial nail removal with the application of a caustic chemical, such as phenol or sodium hydroxide, to the root of the nail in the area removed to prevent regrowth of that part of the nail. Wound care, as with the partial nail removal, must be performed daily for two to three weeks. Other techniques to permanently correct ingrown nails include surgical matrixectomy, radio frequency ablation, and electric or thermal destruction of the nail root.

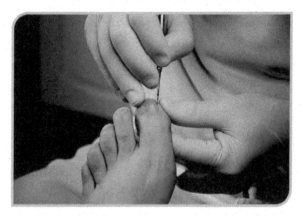

Nonsurgical techniques to manage ingrown nails can be effective in cases where the nail has yet to penetrate the skin around the nail. These include filing the nail edge, packing cotton into the nail grooves, and taping to pull the skin away from the nail. Reducing nail thickness by grinding can help reduce shoe pressure, which can push the nail into the skin. Managing underlying nail pathology such as nail fungus is also helpful, as the thickening and brittleness of the fungal nail can lead to or worsen ingrown nails Noninvasive nail-correction devices are another conservative option for addressing an ingrown nail in its early stages. These devices are applied to the nail and provide a gentle, corrective force that, over time, helps to change the shape of the nail, thus reducing the tendency for it to grow into the skin. The most innovative device of this type today is the Onyfix® system. This employs an acrylic polymer that is applied to the surface of the nail. Once cured with the LED light, the hardened material exerts a corrective force on the nail as it grows. The material will remain on the nail throughout the growth cycle for typically six to eight months. Early results have been good with this device. It is especially useful for those who are not surgical candidates or are needle-phobic.

Occasionally, an underlying bone pathology can cause chronic ingrown toenails. The most common bone abnormality associated with ingrown nails is a bone spur under the nail. These are benign growths of bone and cartilage that form on the top of the end toe bone, the distal phalanx. As these lesions get larger, they can press up under the nail bed and affect the shape of the nail. The curved nail shape and the interaction with the shoe toe box can result in chronic ingrown nails. If suspected, an x-ray examination using a toe isolation technique can help diagnose a bone spur. Because the cartilage part of the lesion is not visible on an x-ray, the lesion could be larger than what appears. Bone spurs are often related to blunt trauma to the toe. Sometimes these lesions can arise without a cause.

Conservative care for this issue consists of wearing shoes with a higher toe box and cushioning the toe with shielding materials such as tubular foam or silicone gel. Surgical removal of a bone spur can be safely performed in an office under local anesthetic, often using minimally invasive techniques through small incisions in the tip of the toe. With a very large lesion, skin plasty (the removal of redundant skin) may be needed to restore the shape of the toe and nail bed area. Occasionally, these procedures require removal of the toenail prior to the procedure. Postoperative care is similar to other forefoot surgical procedures, requiring two to four weeks in a surgical shoe and suture removal after two weeks. Nail regrowth after removal can take six months or more.

NAIL TRAUMA

Trauma to the nail area is a common reason for a visit to the emergency department or doctor's office. Blunt trauma is most often the cause of the injury, either by kicking the foot into something or dropping a heavy object on the toe. The most common resulting issue of blunt toe trauma is blood under the nail, called subungual hematoma. Bleeding under the nail can also be caused by chronic toe trauma, such as ill-fitting footwear. Subungual hematomas can be very painful, often worse than the initial trauma. The trapped fluid has nowhere to go and cannot expand the nail plate. Pressure builds up and pushes into the underlying nail bed, causing pain. Rapid pain relief can be achieved by draining the fluid using a needle inserted under the nail plate from the end. This usually does not require anesthetics. Simple gauze dressing to collect any further drainage may be needed for a few days. A decision on further treatment is based on whether there is an underlying bone injury, such as a fracture. Some patients with subungual hematoma will eventually lose the toenail. A new nail will begin to grow and will eventually push off the old nail, starting from the base of the nail and moving toward the tip of the toe. Loosening nails should be protected from accidental tearing by securing them with tape or an adhesive bandage until the nails are completely loose. Partially detached nails can be removed after a local anesthetic block to remove this annoyance.

Traumatic nail avulsion is a type of trauma where the nail plate is forcefully detached from the nail bed. This can be part of the nail or the entire nail. These injuries will bleed a lot due to the abundant blood supply of the nail bed. You should control bleeding with elevation and a pressure dressing. People taking blood thinners may need to seek medical attention to control bleeding with hemostatic medications.

There is controversy on whether a partial traumatic nail avulsion (removal or detachment) should be completed or if the nail should be left in place to protect the nail bed. My preference is to treat all traumatic nail avulsions as complete and fully remove any partial nail avulsions under a local anesthetic block. This allows for accurate inspection of the nail bed for lacerations, which can then be sutured. Open fractures of the end toe bone can also be ruled out. I find that new nail growth is faster and more even after total nail avulsion versus partial.

Penetrating or sharp trauma to the nail area should be approached in the same manner. Nail removal is often necessary in these situations to fully assess the injury and repair the damage. Nail regrowth after removal can take six to twelve months to return to normal. Injury to the tissues of the nail root area can result in an irregular nail surface, which may be permanent.

For any trauma to the nail area, an x-ray examination should be done to check for fractures of the toe bones. Open fractures should be managed aggressively to prevent bone infection. They should be vigorously cleaned under local anesthetic to remove debris and reduce contamination. Patients must continue good daily wound care until the wound heals in one to three weeks. Reduction and/or fixation of fractures of the end toe bone are not typically needed. Prophylactic antibiotic treatment with a broad-spectrum antibiotic agent should be used for ten to fourteen days or longer. An x-ray should be performed every two weeks to evaluate bone healing and look for signs of bone infection.

Nail unit trauma that results in significant tissue loss may require advanced tissue products or skin grafts to provide for wound closure. Amniotic tissue grafts and bio engineered skin substitutes are options that can be employed in an office setting. Skin grafts, if needed, would have to be performed in a hospital operating room due to the need for anesthesia to obtain the donor tissue, usually from the upper thigh.

Nail irregularity after trauma is common. Many times, irregularity will resolve with nail turnover. In cases of chronic nail plate irregularity, where infectious causes such as fungus have been ruled out, permanent total nail removal can be considered. This can provide symptomatic relief as well as improved cosmetic appearance. Callused skin often forms over the nail bed following permanent nail removal and can look similar to an actual nail. Nail polish can even be applied to this area, although it will not last as long as when on an actual nail.

SYSTEMIC DISEASE AND NAIL CHANGES

Many diseases can cause changes in the appearance and quality of the nail unit. There are entire textbooks dedicated to this subject. Here are some of the most commonly seen diseases in clinical practice.

Nail dystrophy is a term describing nails that are abnormal in appearance. Typically, they can be thick, discolored, and brittle. These nail changes are most often seen in fungal nail infections; systemic conditions can also cause a similar appearance. Nails with this appearance that have repeated negative fungal cultures and/or fail to respond to antifungal therapy should be investigated for underlying conditions, such as psoriasis, lichen planus, Reiter's syndrome, and sarcoidosis. A diagnosis can be made through a patient's history, a full body examination for telltale skin lesions, and a laboratory and microscopic examination of nail and skin biopsies. Managing the underlying condition can help improve the appearance of the nails. Reducing nail thickness can also improve the appearance and reduce symptoms. Softening agents such as urea gel preparations can help improve the nail's condition and appearance, as can taking biotin and vitamin B supplements.

Nail clubbing refers to a change in the shape of the nail and tip of the toe to resemble the end of a club. Clubbed nails are usually associated with pulmonary conditions like COPD and cancer as well as cardiac conditions such as congenital malformations and endocarditis, an infection of the inside lining of the heart.

Spoon-shaped nails describe a nail with a depressed center and upturned edges. Spoon-shaped nails can be seen with iron deficiency anemia, hemochromatosis, lupus, and nail patella syndrome.

Pigmented streaks can be a normal finding in people with deeply pigmented skin. These longitudinal lines are usually regular with straight edges and are of a uniform color. Melanoma skin cancer that affects the nail root area can also present with a pigmented nail streak. Suspicious signs of pigmented nail streaks include irregular edges, a triangular shape with the wider part at the nail root, and color variation. A nail unit biopsy should be done for suspicious nail streaks since early detection is critical in managing this deadly malignancy.

Another longitudinal dark line of the nail unit is called a splinter hemorrhage. These thin, black lines form under the nail and can be mistaken for wood splinters. Splinter hemorrhages are commonly associated with a cardiac condition called subacute bacterial endocarditis (SBE) and are often an early sign of this condition. SBE is an infection of the inner lining of the heart caused by slow-growing bacteria. The heart growths that these infections cause can result in blood clots that can travel to distant sites, commonly resulting in the blockage of nail bed arterioles, which result in splinter hemorrhages. Other causes of splinter hemorrhage-like discoloration are fungal infections, trauma, and psoriasis.

Transverse lines running across the surface of the nail from edge to edge that are indented are usually benign. They are often related to trauma or severe systemic diseases that temporarily disrupt the nail root growth. These lines will grow out with normal nail growth in six to twelve months. However, white transverse lines without a depression can however, can be an indication of toxic exposure, particularly from arsenic.

Yellow nail syndrome is a rare condition where the fingernails and toenails become yellowed. The nails can be thick as well, and this condition can be misdiagnosed as a fungal infection. The exact cause of yellow nail syndrome is not clear. It is thought to be related to lymphedema, a buildup of fluid in the tissue of the extremities. Hereditary conditions and prior infections such as cellulitis can predispose a person to lymphedema due to injury to the lymphatic vessels that carry the fluid back from the extremities to the central circulatory system. Treatment of yellow nail syndrome is usually palliative and employs methods such as reducing thickness and discoloration through electric grinding and the application of nail conditioners such as urea gel.

Blue toenails can occur due to a number of conditions. Blue discoloration of the nails and digits is usually associated with high levels of deoxygenated hemoglobin in the peripheral circulation. Lung conditions such as COPD, asthma, and pulmonary embolism can cause someone to have blue nails. Cardiac conditions such as congestive heart failure and congenital heart defects are another cause of blue nails. They can also be related to blood abnormalities such as methemoglobinemia, polycythemia vera, and carbon monoxide poisoning.

THREE

Skin Conditions

Many foot and ankle specialists focus on the musculoskeletal conditions of patients. Skin and nail conditions, however, are some of the most common complaints that patients have with their feet. This chapter will describe the most common skin conditions likely to be seen in the lower extremities and some effective treatment options.

COMMON SKIN CONDITIONS

CORNS AND CALLUSES

Corns and calluses are likely the number one skin condition seen in lower-extremity practices. The profession of podiatry has its roots in providing nonsurgical care for this annoying and often painful condition. Corns and calluses are discrete keratotic lesions, meaning they are composed of compressed layers of keratin, the outer layer of skin. This layer has no living cells and no nerve endings, thus the lack of pain when removed sharply. Pain from these lesions is typically due to the pressure from weight-bearing or from shoes that press the lesions into the underlying soft tissue, which has nerve endings. These lesions typically form in areas with frequent pressure or friction and are the body's attempt at protection. Corns and calluses are basically the same condition. The term corn usually refers to a smaller, more concentrated lesion, where callus is often used to refer to broader, larger lesions. The terms are often used interchangeably. These commonly form on the tops of the toes, the tips of the toes, between the toes, the bottom of the foot under the metatarsals, and on the edge of the heel. They can arise anywhere there is an underlying bony prominence if it is rubbing in the shoe or on the bottom of the foot. A diagnosis is made through visual inspection and is confirmed by reducing the lesions.

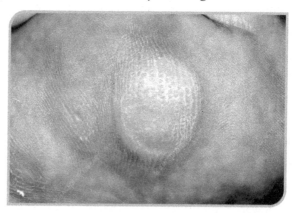

Treatment of corns and calluses is initiated with the reduction of their thickness to reduce pressure on underlying structures. This is commonly performed by podiatrists using a sharp surgical blade or a grinding machine. Chemical reduction using urea or salicylic acid compounds are another option, though results are slower to achieve. Padding the areas to reduce shoe or weight-bearing pressure can also help control symptoms. It is essential to identify and manage underlying structural and/or biomechanical abnormalities for long-term relief. This often involves shoe gear modification, foot orthotics or bracing, and potentially surgical procedures to correct deformities or reduce bony prominences. It is common to need periodic reduction of recurrent lesions if underlying forces are not adequately controlled. Typical intervals are one to three months apart.

VERRUCAE

Verrucae, also known as warts, are skin lesions that are caused by variants of the human papilloma virus. Warts are commonly confused with corns or calluses. At first glance, they can look similar due to the increased keratotic layer formed over and around the wart due to pressure from weight-bearing. Upon reduction of the keratin layer, it can be seen that the wart extends to the deeper levels of the skin. Interruption of skin lines is a common diagnostic sign, as are the small capillaries that feed the wart tissue, which show pinpoint bleeding on reduction beneath the keratotic layer. Smaller verrucae that are under three millimeters often have not developed much of a capillary bed yet and can therefore be readily mistaken for a corn, especially if they are near a bony prominence. Verrucae on the bottom of the foot are termed plantar warts, referring to the plantar or bottom surface of the foot. Warts on other areas of the foot are termed common warts or verruca vulgaris. They are usually diagnosed through clinical examination. Occasionally, a biopsy may be needed for definitive diagnosis.

Verrucae have been treated in a number of ways throughout history. In modern medicine, treatments include topical debriding agents such as salicylic acid, blistering agents, drying agents, immunotherapy, and surgical removal.

There are no oral antiviral medications or vaccines that have been developed for this form of the human papilloma virus. An off-label use of a common antacid medication, cimetidine, can be a helpful adjunctive therapy, especially with children. It is thought that this medication somehow modulates the immune response to the virus. I have had success with this treatment, even as monotherapy, in children as young as three. Cimetidine can be obtained in a liquid elixir, which is helpful when treating younger patients.

I have used many combinations of treatments for verrucae throughout my years of practice. I have found the most effective method to be the combination of a chemical blistering agent followed by laser photodynamic therapy. This technique has proved highly effective, even with large and/ or multiple lesions. After debridement of the keratotic layer, the blistering agent, Cantharone®, is applied to the lesion and covered for twenty-four hours. The area can then be washed and re-dressed if needed for protection. One week later, the blistered area is debrided and a dye solution of methylene blue is applied to the area and allowed to dry. The area is then treated with laser energy at low levels for two minutes in each area. The laser energy interacts with the dye molecules in the target tissue to cause cell death, eliminating any remaining abnormal tissue. Large or multiple lesions may require additional treatments. Recurrence is rare after resolution following this technique.

Verrucae that fail to respond to conservative efforts should be considered for biopsy to rule out a malignancy. Verrucae are contagious, so care should be taken to avoid spreading them to other people. Moist environments such as bathtubs, showers, and pool decks are common areas where they are spread. Sanitization of these surfaces with a diluted bleach solution can be effective. Avoid sharing footwear with others, and allow shoes to dry fully between wearings.

TINEA PEDIS

Tinea pedis, commonly called athlete's foot, is a fungal infection of the outer skin layers of the foot. The most common type of fungus to cause tinea pedis is a dermatophyte. Two common areas of occurrence of tinea pedis are between the toes and on the sole of the foot. Fungal infections between the toes tend to be moist, whereas fungal infections on the soles tend to be dry. Typically, peeling of the outer skin layers is seen in patchy areas along with small, dry blisters. The most common symptom of tinea pedis is itching, which can lead to skin abrasions from scratching. These abrasions can become secondarily infected by bacteria, causing abscesses or cellulitis. Tinea pedis is usually diagnosed by clinical evaluation. Laboratory evaluation of skin scrapings may also be performed to help identify unusual organisms and is especially helpful in treating resistant cases.

Treatment using topical antifungal preparations for two to four weeks is usually curative. In severe infections and those not responding to topical treatments, oral antifungal medications may be needed for one to two weeks. Recurrence of tinea pedis is common, especially in susceptible

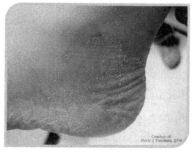

individuals. Prevention of recurrence revolves around moisture management and reducing exposure to fungal organisms.

Fungi thrive in dark, moist environments like the inside of shoes, so footwear must be dried thoroughly between wearings. Dry your feet well after washing, especially between the toes. When applied regularly, an antifungal powder or spray can absorb moisture and reduce fungal organisms. If using moisturizers on the feet, avoid applying between the toes, as these areas can get too moist, increasing the risk of a fungal infection. People with recurrent fungal infections should consider sanitizing all footwear regularly by using a commercial spray or ultraviolet sterilizer.

HYPERKERATOSIS

Hyperkeratosis is a group of skin conditions that result in skin that is excessively dry and scaly. The scaling can become very thick, especially around the edges of the foot. The thickened areas can develop cracks that can extend into the deeper skin layers and increase the potential for a bacterial infection. Mild hyperkeratosis can be treated with a variety of over-the-counter moisturizers applied one to two times daily. More severe cases may require more potent softening agents, such as urea preparations in concentrations of 40 to 50 percent. Apply these to the affected areas two to four times a day. Sharp reduction of heavy scaling by a medical professional can also be helpful at relieving symptoms. Areas with full-thickness skin cracks can be treated with topical corticosteroid preparations two to four times daily for two to four weeks.

ECZEMA

Eczema, or dermatitis, is another common keratotic skin condition. Dermatitis starts with inflammation in the deeper skin layers and can develop thickening of the outer layers with scaling, peeling, and cracking. Itching is a common complaint. Scratching can contribute to the thickening of the skin. Microscopic examination of skin scrapings and occasionally a full-thickness skin biopsy may be necessary to differentiate dermatitis from tinea pedis. There are several potential causes of dermatitis, the most common being exposure to toxins (contact dermatitis), allergy (atopic dermatitis), and family background (hereditary dermatitis). The treatment for this uses topical corticosteroid preparations of various potencies to address any underlying causes. Exfoliation of keratotic areas with topical urea preparations and/or sharp debridement can help improve symptoms. Non-responding cases may require a short course of oral corticosteroids or a biologic agent such as dupilumab.

PSORIASIS

Psoriasis is an autoimmune skin condition that causes the skin cells to multiply at much faster rates, causing red, raised, scaly lesions to form. The feet are not the most common part of the body for psoriasis to present, but they are not spared. Psoriasis lesions are more common on the top of the foot and legs. Plantar surface psoriatic plaques, when they do form, can be painful to walk on. Psoriasis can cause the toenails to become brittle and thickened, appearing similar to fungal toenails. A diagnosis is usually made by clinical symptoms and the appearance of the lesions. A skin biopsy may be needed to confirm diagnosis or differentiate this from other skin conditions. Many different treatments have been used for psoriasis over the years. Examples include coal tar, UV light therapy, vitamin A derivatives, corticosteroids, photodynamic therapy, immunosuppressive agents, and biologic agents.

NEOPLASIA

Malignant skin tumors are rare in the lower extremity. The majority of abnormal skin growths are benign, or nonthreatening. The most common benign skin growths are nevi, or moles. These dark-colored lesions are collections of cells with high levels of the skin pigment melanin. Nevi are typically small and regular in shape and color. Warts can also fall into this category of skin tumors. As noted above, they are caused by an infection of the skin cells. Another common skin tumor is a dermal fibroma. These are benign growths of fibrous tissue in the dermis, the deepest skin layer.

These flesh-colored lesions are usually small and isolated. They are commonly located in the skin surrounding the nails. A lesion that has a similar appearance is the neurofibroma. This lesion is composed of neural tissues as well as fibrous tissue. Although benign, neurofibromatosis can result in multiple lesions all over the body. Actinic, or solar, keratosis is another common skin growth. These small, raised, flesh-colored lesions are thought to be caused by sun exposure. Benign skin tumors tend to be slow growing and do not spread locally or to distant areas. All benign skin growths should be monitored over time to look for changes that could be worrisome for malignant change. Any skin lesion that has changed considerably should be examined microscopically. Biopsy can usually provide an accurate diagnosis of the skin tumor to guide further treatment.

The most common malignant skin tumors that occur on the feet are malignant melanoma and squamous cell carcinoma. Both can be very aggressive and spread locally and to distant areas, including the lungs, liver, and brain. Early suspicion and microscopic evaluation are key to preventing morbidity and mortality from these tumors. Characteristics of melanoma that raise suspicion revolve around the ABCs. A stands for *area*. Lesions larger than six millimeters are considered suspicious. B stands for *border irregularity*. Benign nevi tend to have smooth borders. Irregularity of the edges of a pigmented lesion raises suspicion of malignancy. C stands for *color variation*. Benign skin lesions tend to be uniform in color. Variations in color throughout a skin lesion are a suspicious sign. Squamous cell carcinoma can be difficult to identify clinically. It often presents as a nonhealing wound or ulceration on the extremities. Any wound that fails to heal with adequate wound care should be considered suspicious. On rare occasions, chronic wounds, such as diabetic foot ulcers or pressure ulcers can undergo malignant degeneration and become cancerous, leading to squamous cell carcinoma. As above, stalled wound healing should be considered suspicious for malignant change.

FOUR
Peripheral Neuropathy

Neuropathy is a medical term that describes nerve abnormality. Nerve tissue allows communication within the body using electrical and chemical signals, helping to govern all bodily functions. In the human body, the nervous system is divided into the central nervous system, which includes the brain and spinal cord, and the peripheral nervous system, which is all the nerve tissue outside of the central nervous system. There is an intimate interconnection between the central and peripheral nervous systems. This chapter will focus on conditions that affect the peripheral nervous system, termed peripheral neuropathy.

Peripheral neuropathy is a common condition that affects an estimated twenty million people in the United States, causing symptoms and complications that range from mild annoyance to severe mobility disturbances to life-threatening. The three main types of peripheral nerves in the body are sensory, motor, and autonomic. Sensory nerves allow us to perceive the world around us—pain perception, temperature perception, and joint position sense are examples of sensory nerve functions. Motor nerves allow our body to signal muscles to contract, allowing us to move about. Autonomic nerves control other non-volitional body functions such as sweating, blood flow, breathing, and digestion.

Peripheral neuropathies can be further classified into mononeuropathies (those affecting single nerves), or polyneuropathies (those affecting multiple nerves). Polyneuropathy is much more common than mononeuropathy.

Although it is not a direct result of the aging process, neuropathy is rare in people under forty. It is estimated that 8 percent of Americans over the age of fifty-five are affected by some form of neuropathy.

Over one hundred causes of neuropathy have been described in medical literature. Neuropathy is the number one most common complication of diabetes, affecting 50 percent of diabetics at some point in their disease. Some other common causes we see in clinical practice are spinal nerve compression/stenosis, chemotherapy exposure, alcoholism, toxin exposure (such as lead), infections (such as Lyme disease, herpes, and HIV), autoimmune disorders (such as Guillain-Barré syndrome), nutritional deficiencies, and inflammatory conditions. Neuropathies with no definitive cause are termed idiopathic neuropathies.

Nerves conduct electrical and chemical signals throughout the body. Like the electrical wiring in our homes, most peripheral nerves are wrapped in an insulating tissue called myelin. Many neuropathies result in a degradation of the myelin sheath, resulting in inefficient transmission of nerve impulses. These conditions are termed demyelinating neuropathies. Some neuropathies affect the nerve cell itself, leading to inefficient nerve impulses. These are termed axonal neuropathies. Inefficient nerve impulse transmission results in abnormal body functions, leading to the signs and symptoms of neuropathy.

Peripheral neuropathy can present with or without symptoms. Sensory symptoms can include numbness, tingling, burning, itching, and other abnormal sensations. Neuropathic pain can be relatively mild or severe enough to require narcotic pain medications. It can also cause balance difficulties due to loss of position sensation. Motor symptoms can include weakness of the extremities and loss of coordination. Motor nerve dysfunction can also contribute to balance issues. Autonomic nerve symptoms can include excessive skin dryness and cold feet and hands. People without symptoms often present to lower-extremity providers only after they suffer from a complication of neuropathy, such as a foot ulcer, Charcot foot, or an unnoticed injury. It is important to identify asymptomatic neuropathy patients to prevent future complications from neuropathy. This is why an annual foot screening that includes vascular and neurological examinations is recommended for all diabetic patients.

DIAGNOSIS

Diagnosis of peripheral neuropathy is usually made through a comprehensive history and physical examination. A history of symptoms like those above provides a clue to the diagnosis. A neurological examination should include sensory, motor, and autonomic testing.

Sensory testing usually includes vibratory sensation, joint position sensation, temperature discrimination, sharp/dull discrimination, two-point discrimination, and protective pressure sensation using the ten-gram monofilament test. Motor testing should include deep tendon reflexes, muscle-power testing, and gait analysis. Balance can be evaluated using postural sway measurements, single-leg stance testing, and force platforms. Autonomic dysfunction is the most difficult to test for. For that, skin temperature measurement and moisture meters can be helpful as well as an observation for skin dryness.

Electrophysiologic testing, such as nerve conduction velocity and electromyogram, are not good screening tests because changes in these measurements often occur much later in the progression of peripheral neuropathy. They can, however, be helpful in determining the type of neuropathy, demyelinating or axonal, and/or the presence and location of compression neuropathies. Epidermal nerve fiber density testing is a sensitive test that uses a small sample of skin to determine the number of small nerve fibers in the epidermis. This can help confirm the diagnosis, especially in those who produce negative electrophysiologic test results but have positive signs and symptoms. It can also gauge the effectiveness of treatments discussed in the next section.

TREATMENT

Controlling causative conditions such as diabetes, alcoholism, and infections are an important starting point. Most conventional medical treatments for neuropathy focus on symptom management. Pain is the most commonly treated symptom of neuropathy. A variety of classes of medication have been used for neuropathic pain with varying results. These include analgesics, anti-inflammatories, narcotics, anticonvulsants, and antidepressants. Topical anesthetics, anti-inflammatories, and capsaicin preparations have also been used with varying results. None of these medications have been shown to improve nerve function or reverse the signs and symptoms of neuropathy.

Nutritional support of the nerves and electrical nerve stimulation have been proven to improve nerve function and reverse signs and symptoms of various neuropathies.

Correcting nutritional deficiencies revealed in a laboratory examination is necessary for general and nerve health. The modern diet has several common deficiencies, including vitamin D, magnesium, zinc, and essential fatty acids. A vitamin B12 deficiency can even cause neuropathy. Aside from deficiencies, certain nutritional supplements have been shown to help improve nerve function in general: B vitamins, particularly B1, B6, and B12, can provide support to nerve healing. Alpha lipoic acid, a substance that has been studied and used extensively in Europe to manage a number of medical conditions including liver disease and poisoning, has been shown to help reverse the nerve damage from neuropathy. Prescription supplements such as Metanx® include versions of the three B vitamins mentioned. Prescriptive supplements can be expensive and may not be covered by health insurance plans. Quality nonprescription supplements can be obtained from a number of sources. Look for manufacturers that are GMP certified and use independent testing for verification.

Compression neuropathies can be managed with surgical release of the entrapped or compressed nerve. Common areas of entrapment in the lower extremity include the metatarsal area, the top of the mid-foot, the tarsal tunnel area on the inside of the ankle, the fibular neck area (which is just below the outside of the knee), the sciatic notch (which is under the gluteal muscles), and below the lumbar spine. Compression neuropathies can occur at the same time as other neuropathies. Removing the compression on the nerve with a surgical release can usually help the nerve recover from the underlying neuropathy as well by allowing improved blood and nutrient flow. Ablation or destruction of the offending nerve can be attempted in cases resistant to all other treatments. This is most appropriate for mononeuropathies, as they only affect a single or small number of nerves.

Physical therapy can be helpful with the management of the sequelae, or secondary effects, of neuropathies including weakness, balance problems, joint contractures, and gait disturbances. Physical medicine modalities can be used to manage neuropathic pain as well as infrared light therapy, class 4 laser treatment. Various forms of electrical stimulation have been shown to be helpful at reducing neuropathic pain.

There is a specific electrical therapy technique that has been proven to help improve nerve health and function as well as reduce symptoms. This technique is termed electric signal therapy (EST). The original device designed for this treatment is the Neurogenx 4000 device. For years, peripheral nerve damage was thought to be irreversible. But more and more scientific and medical research is indicating that in many cases of neuropathy, nerve tissue may be dormant rather than dead, and it is possible that function may be restored with proper stimulation and signaling. The Neurogenx 4000 device is the first device that has been clinically shown to improve nerve function using electrical energy. EST is a more sophisticated treatment than the familiar transcutaneous electrical nerve stimulation (TENS) and electrical muscle stimulation (EMS) types of stimulation. EST with Neurogenx uses a microprocessor to deliver biosimilar electrical energy to the body. The waveform of this energy is nearly identical to the human body's own nerve impulses. This waveform better stimulates the chemical signaling within the nerve tissue, allowing for better cell interconnection and permitting the flow of nutrients within the nerve tissue. The microprocessor changes the frequency at regular intervals, which prevents the body from adapting to the stimulation during the treatment cycle, further enhancing effectiveness. EST stimulation creates changes within the nerve cells themselves, including increasing metabolism, normalizing pH balance, allowing fluid and waste product removal, signaling nerve cell growth, and improving efficiency of nerve impulse transmission. The end result is improved nerve function and reduction of the symptoms of neuropathy.

EST is usually effective on its own. In some cases with a slow response to this therapy, combining EST with chemical nerve block can improve the effectiveness of the treatments. Integrated nerve block uses injections of small amounts of local anesthetic agents around the target nerves followed by EST treatment. Local anesthetics work by causing a sustained depolarization of the nerve, similar to the main effect of EST. The combination of the two techniques can improve effectiveness in difficult cases compared with each on its own. The typical protocol for EST is twice weekly for eight weeks. Integrated nerve blocks would be performed at every other session, if indicated.

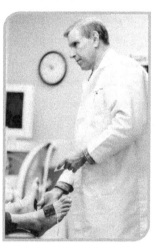

Most patients have symptom improvement after a few sessions, though neuropathies that are more profound may require longer treatment plans. Patients with progressive neuropathies may require maintenance treatment weekly to monthly to maintain the improvement. I have been using this technology in my practice for five years and have seen some remarkable results. Over 80 percent of patients treated with this technology report a significant improvement in the signs and symptoms of peripheral neuropathy. Improvements can often be seen within three to four treatment sessions. Improvements in nerve health can be measured through repeat epidermal nerve fiber density biopsy following treatment. Repeat testing has shown increases in nerve fiber density as much as 700 percent. Significant reduction in pain scores are also seen, and improvements in balance and walking ability lead to a better quality of life for neuropathy patients.

Advancements in medicine and technology have provided hope for those who suffer from the effects of peripheral neuropathy. Continued research in the diagnosis and treatment of nerve conditions is needed, as there are many who suffer from these conditions.

FIVE

Diabetes and the Feet

Diabetes mellitus is a medical condition affecting millions of people worldwide. Its prevalence is increasing every year. Reasons for the explosion in the numbers of people with this condition are in debate. The widespread adoption of the so-called western diet, which is high in carbohydrates, processed foods, and unhealthy oils, along with declining physical activity levels in modern societies are surely contributory factors. When someone has diabetes, their body does not properly regulate their blood glucose level. Persistently elevated blood glucose and insulin levels cause damaging effects on the body.

There are two main types of diabetes mellitus. Type 1 diabetes typically begins in childhood and is a result of the body's inability to produce the hormone insulin, which regulates blood glucose. The prevailing theory about the cause of this is that an autoimmune response affects the insulin-producing cells in the pancreas organ, stopping insulin production. People with type 1 diabetes must have insulin injections to survive. Type 2 diabetes typically occurs in adulthood and is strongly associated with diet and obesity. Early stages of type 2 diabetes are marked by higher than normal insulin levels as the body attempts to store excess dietary calories. With persistent high insulin levels, the body's cells become resistant to the effect of insulin, and cell uptake of glucose is slowed, leading to high blood glucose. Type 2 diabetes is usually treated with various oral medications to lower blood glucose levels. When oral medications fail to control blood sugar levels, insulin injections may be a necessary part of treatment.

Persistently elevated blood glucose and insulin levels have many negative effects on the body, resulting in many complications. Peripheral neuropathy and peripheral vascular disease are the main complications that affect the lower extremities.

PERIPHERAL NEUROPATHY

Neuropathy is a term referring to nerve dysfunction. Peripheral nerves are those outside of the brain and spinal cord. These nerves connect the skin, muscle, and sensory and digestive organs to the brain and spinal cord. The nerves that serve the lower extremities have sensory, motor, and autonomic functions. Sensory nerves help perceive the world around us; motor nerves help the body move; and autonomic nerves control blood flow and sweating. Diabetic peripheral neuropathy (DPN) affects all nerve types in the extremities.

Elevated blood glucose levels cause direct damage to nerve tissue and lead to vascular disease of the small blood vessels that supply the nerves.

Symptoms of neuropathy include numbness, tingling, burning, or diffuse pain. Balance issues can be a sign of peripheral nerve dysfunction, and it can cause excessive skin dryness. The most dangerous complication that can occur with peripheral neuropathy is a loss of protective sensation because it can allow trauma to go unnoticed, leading to skin breakdown and ulceration. Ulcerations can then lead to infections of skin, soft tissue, and bone. Foot ulceration is the leading cause of lower-extremity amputation in diabetic patients.

Prompt, skilled treatment by a lower-extremity specialist is needed to manage neuropathy. This challenging condition is diagnosed primarily through history and physical examination. Sensory loss in DPN is usually symmetrical and starts from the toes and spreads upward. Physical testing of the various sensory perceptions in the lower extremities can help to identify and quantify the neuropathy. Protective sensation is determined using the ten-gram monofilament test, where a small nylon filament is pressed onto various parts of the feet to determine whether the patient can perceive the pressure of the filament. Electrophysiological nerve testing such as nerve conduction velocity (NCV) and electromyogram (EMG) often do not show changes until diabetic neuropathy is in its advanced stages, so they are not useful screening tests. They can, however, be helpful for ruling out other causes of neuropathy. Finally, an epidermal nerve fiber density test can help identify small fiber neuropathy. This test involves a skin biopsy with special stains used to reveal the nerve tissue. The nerve fibers are counted and compared to normal numbers.

Treatment of neuropathy starts with tight control of blood glucose levels to slow down damage to the nerves. Symptoms can be managed using a variety of topical and oral medications. Unfortunately, this is where treatment usually ends in the healthcare system. Fortunately, there are therapeutic alternatives that have been shown to restore nerve function. EST is one such modality. This technique involves the application of electrical energy to the body in biosimilar waveforms using a computerized program. This energy effectively wakes up dormant nerves and improves their function. Many patients who have been treated with this technique have had significant reductions in symptoms and improvement in balance and function. Nutritional support of the nerves is also critical for success. Laser stimulation of the extremities has also been shown to help. Higher-energy, class 4 medical laser devices are the most effective for managing neuropathy symptoms.

Entrapment and/or compression of nerves in various anatomic areas can contribute to the symptoms of neuropathy. Nerves affected by diabetes are more prone to damage by compression than healthy nerves. This is believed to be due to intraneural swelling. In cases where compression neuropathy is complicating DPN, decompression surgery can improve local nutrient flow within the nerve, permitting recovery to proceed. The most common nerve entrapment in the lower extremity is the posterior tibial nerve in an area called the tarsal tunnel. This area is behind and below the inside anklebone. Other potential sites of compression include the deep peroneal nerve on the top of the mid-foot and the common peroneal nerve just below the outside of the knee.

PERIPHERAL ARTERIAL DISEASE

Peripheral arterial disease (PAD) is a condition of the arteries in the extremities in which blood flow is reduced due to narrowing of the inside of the arteries because of atherosclerotic plaques. Atherosclerosis occurs earlier and is more widespread in diabetic patients than in the general population. Symptoms of PAD include coldness of the toes and feet, leg cramps with walking, pain while at rest, and nonhealing wounds. Redness of the skin when the feet are on the floor with whiteness of the skin on elevation is a clinical sign of PAD, which is diagnosed through physical examination along with vascular testing. Noninvasive Doppler waveform testing and segmental blood pressures are effective at identifying and quantifying PAD.

Percutaneous angiography, a minimally invasive surgical and diagnostic technique, can pinpoint blockages and allow the vascular specialist to remove plaques and open arteries with stents. Arteries that cannot be opened by these techniques may need an open surgical bypass to salvage the limb. Good communication between the vascular specialist and lower-extremity specialist is needed to manage vascular-related foot complications. In all cases of PAD, exercising the leg muscles is important to help the body form new blood vessels around blockages. This is known as collateral circulation. Medications to improve blood flow are limited, but pentoxifylline is an agent that increases the flexibility of blood cells, allowing them to move through narrow arteries easier. This can be helpful in early stages of PAD. Nitroglycerine paste applied to the skin of the toes can also cause a temporary increase in blood flow, reducing symptoms. But most importantly, patients must manage the underlying medical conditions that contribute to PAD such as lipid abnormalities, high blood pressure, and diabetes.

FOOT ULCERS

CAUSES

Foot ulcers are one of the most dangerous complications caused by diabetes. A foot ulcer is a wound through the skin, exposing deep structures such as fat, muscle, tendon, and bone. Foot ulcers are the leading cause of amputations of

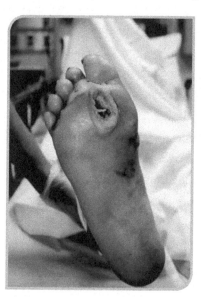

the lower extremities in patients with diabetes. They usually begin with some type of trauma to the skin. This can range from penetration from a foreign body, like stepping on a sharp object, to simple shoe pressure on a bony prominence. Many foot ulcers are related to neuropathy. Trauma can go unnoticed because of

the loss of protective sensation. This lets repetitive trauma occur that exceeds the repair capability of the body. Tissue injury and breakdown occur, leaving an opening in the skin barrier. Infectious microorganisms can then gain access to the inside of the body, leading to soft-tissue and bone infections. Severe vascular compromise from PAD is another potential cause of ulceration. In this condition, blood flow cannot adequately provide tissues with nutrients for repair from trauma, resulting in tissue breakdown. Abrupt stoppage of blood flow to an area by a blood clot in a small artery can also cause an ulceration. Patients with both neuropathy and PAD are at the highest risk for ulceration and amputation. Foot deformities such as bunions, hammertoes, plantar-flexed metatarsals, and flatfeet can contribute to foot ulcers by causing abnormal pressure areas during weight-bearing activities. Posterior heel ulcers are a risk for bedbound patients with neuropathy and/or PAD due to prolonged pressure on the heel from the bed.

EVALUATION

Foot ulcerations are usually staged or graded based on the size and depth of the tissue injury and whether there is an infection and/or PAD or frank gangrene. The greatest risk posed by foot ulcerations is the potential for infections from invading microorganisms. Infections can have both limb-threatening and life-threatening complications that require prompt and aggressive management.

Evaluation of foot ulcers involves visual inspection and physical probing of the wound with sterile instruments to assess its depth. Underlying medical and orthopedic conditions should be identified and managed. An x-ray evaluation can help identify underlying bony deformities and uncover signs of bone infection, although x-ray changes due to bone infection are usually not apparent for two to four weeks from the start of the infection. As such, earlier diagnoses often require an MRI, as it is more sensitive to identifying early bone changes. It can also help identify soft-tissue abscesses and anatomically localize infections for surgical planning. Nuclear medicine scans are another sensitive test for bone infections; however, they lack the anatomic clarity of an MRI.

TREATMENT

The key to treating foot ulcerations is to identify and manage the underlying causative and contributory conditions. The most important areas to address are blood sugar control, correction of nutritional deficiencies, relief from repetitive trauma, management of musculoskeletal deformities, and restoration of compromised blood flow. The most advanced wound treatment techniques are doomed to failure without addressing these and any other contributing condition. Lower-extremity practitioners address the underlying musculoskeletal problems that cause pressure areas and repetitive trauma. To do that, they recommend shoe modification, orthotics, bracing, walking boots, casting, and corrective surgery when necessary. Patient adherence to pressure-reducing techniques is essential to the success of any wound care program. The best off-loading treatment will not be effective if not used by the patient.

Medicare enacted the so-called diabetic shoe bill several years ago. This benefit allows diabetic patients with neuropathy and/or vascular impairment with certain foot deformities to receive one pair of extra-depth footwear and three pairs of accommodative insoles each year as a covered benefit. A letter from the doctor managing the patient's diabetes certifying the patient's diabetic status is required, along with a diabetic foot assessment by a lower-extremity specialist, to be maintained as part of the necessary documentation. There are many different brands and styles of shoes that qualify as extra depth for this program. It is best to consult with a qualified lower-extremity specialist who is knowledgeable about footwear and the particulars of this program. Other insurance carriers may also cover depth inlay footwear and insoles for diabetic patients with neuropathy and other conditions.

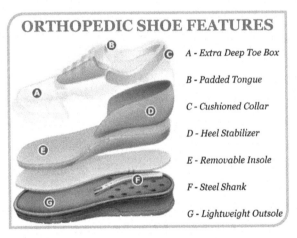

ORTHOPEDIC SHOE FEATURES

A - *Extra Deep Toe Box*

B - *Padded Tongue*

C - *Cushioned Collar*

D - *Heel Stabilizer*

E - *Removable Insole*

F - *Steel Shank*

G - *Lightweight Outsole*

Total-contact casting is one of the most effective ways to off-load a foot wound on the bottom of the foot while allowing the patient to walk. This technique involves applying a well-molded plaster cast to the foot and leg with a relief built in for the ulcerated area. The casts are left in place for one to two weeks at a time, depending on the nature of the wound and the amount of drainage. Occasionally, the cast material over the wound can be removed to create a window for wound care and monitoring. Application of a total-contact cast is time consuming and requires a high level of skill to be a successful treatment modality. An alternative to the total-contact cast can be created using an off-the-shelf controlled ankle motion (CAM) walking boot with fiberglass casting tape applied to the outside to create a non-removable device.

Once underlying factors are adequately managed, good wound care should allow for healing. Patients and caregivers can often be instructed on how to perform dressing changes at home. Sometimes, skilled nursing wound care is needed, which can be provided at home by a visiting nurse service. Long-standing wounds have the tendency to slow or stop the healing process. The goal of wound management is to keep the wound in an acute healing state. This is accomplished by skilled wound care in the office setting. Sharp removal of surrounding calluses and nonviable tissue from the wound using sterile instruments helps to maintain this acute wound state. Wound care should be performed weekly. Good wound care can also reduce the bio burden, which is the number of microorganisms that can lead to infection if left unchecked. Clinically infected wounds should be treated with topical and oral antibiotics until signs of infection have resolved. If necessary, a wound culture using advanced DNA techniques can identify the organisms in the wound and uncover a resistant organism that may need special treatment.

Wounds that fail to progress within four weeks of good wound care may need advanced wound treatments. Laser light stimulation has been shown to be helpful in assisting with wound healing. Low energy applied using wavelengths of 860 and 980 nanometers has been shown to stimulate the wound tissue, increasing local tissue metabolism and decreasing healing time. Becaplermin (brand name Regranex®) is a topical growth factor product that has been shown to reduce healing time in diabetic ulcers. This gel is applied to the wound surface daily when dressings are changed. The gel must be kept refrigerated to maintain its effectiveness. Advanced tissue products can also be used when wounds aren't healing. These tissues have a number of growth factors and cellular products that the body can use to help wound healing. The most commonly employed are donated amniotic tissue products, which are obtained from screened donors during childbirth. The tissues are processed in several ways to preserve them for later use. These tissues have a number of growth factors and cellular products that the body can use to help wound healing. These products are typically applied weekly for eight to ten applications, as needed. For wounds that fail to heal despite the use of advanced tissue products, surgical management may be needed to achieve closure. Skin grafts and tissue flaps are plastic surgery techniques that can be used to close foot wounds of various shapes and sizes. Tissue can be obtained locally from near the wound or from distant sites. A high level of skill and experience is needed to utilize skin grafts and flaps for foot wound closure. The main benefit of skin grafts and flaps is that they utilize the patient's own tissue, allowing for better incorporation and healing than with donor tissue. The downside is that the site where the graft or flap is taken from becomes a wound that also needs to heal.

Every effort is made to obtain tissue from areas with good blood supply and from non-weight-bearing areas whenever possible.

CHARCOT FOOT

Charcot foot, also called neuroarthropathy, is a condition that results in spontaneous dislocation of foot and ankle joints, leading to the collapse of the foot structure. This can result in major bony deformities and prominences that can be subject to abnormally high pressure or friction with weight-bearing and wearing shoes, which can lead to skin breakdown and ulceration. Fortunately, this potentially devastating condition is uncommon.

The exact cause of this condition has yet to be clarified. Sensory and motor nerve dysfunctions are certainly contributory, allowing repetitive injuries to occur and go unnoticed. Autonomic nerve dysfunction is thought to cause an abnormal increase in blood flow to the bone beneath the joint surface, leading to bone mineral loss and weakening of the bone. The weakened bone is not able to resist repetitive trauma, leading to microfractures beneath the joint surface, which can contribute to joint collapse and bone fragmentation. The collapsed Charcot foot is difficult to walk on without bracing or custom footwear. Doctors may attempt major reconstructive surgical procedures to fuse the affected joints in patients with adequate blood supply and stable health conditions, but these procedures have high risks of complications and a lengthy recovery period. Preventing the collapse of a Charcot foot is more ideal.

Early diagnosis and intervention is necessary to prevent a collapsed Charcot foot. Immobilization and non-weight-bearing are required for one to two months to allow the acute inflammatory phase of Charcot to resolve. Doctors need a high index of suspicion (in other words, a high awareness of possible underlying illnesses) to make an early diagnosis of Charcot foot because the swelling and increased temperature of the area can often be confused with infections like cellulitis or other conditions such as deep vein thrombosis or gout. Joint-area swelling with increased temperature accompanied by extreme pain, even in those with profound neuropathy, can be an indicator of early Charcot.

Without adequate treatment during the early phase, joint dislocation and bone fragmentation will occur, leading to foot structure collapse. Eventually, the body will begin to heal the fragmentation and dislocation in a phase termed consolidation. In this phase, the joints restabilize but in positions of deformity. Once consolidation has completed, the patient enters a quiescent, or inactive, phase. Patients who have had Charcot attacks are always at risk for repeated attacks. The consolidated, deformed foot is also at high risk for skin ulceration due to abnormal pressure areas. Custom orthotics, shoes, and bracing are needed to reduce pressure on bony prominences to prevent ulceration. Again, surgical intervention may be necessary in those patients who have continued ulceration despite the use of these conservative techniques.

Prophylactic foot surgery is the term used for surgery performed to correct a deformity with the goal of reducing pressure from shoes or weight-bearing that has or may lead to ulceration. In patients without neuropathy, pain is largely used as a criterion for determining whether surgery is necessary. Most foot deformities can be painless in those with peripheral neuropathy yet can pose an even greater risk to their health and well-being. In all patients, surgical management should only be considered for those who have failed all conservative methods of prevention of ulceration. Adequate blood supply and stable medical status are prerequisites for considering surgical care. There are a number of surgical procedures that can be safely performed in an office or outpatient surgical suite using local anesthesia. They can make a profound improvement on a patient's ability to wear shoes and/or braces. Examples include toe tendon releases, bone spur removal, hammertoe correction, bunion correction, and metatarsal surgery. Major rearfoot or ankle procedures need to be performed in a hospital and usually require general anesthesia and possibly a hospital stay.

The foot complications of diabetes are a challenge for both the patient and clinician to manage. Teamwork between all parties involved in the patient care, including the patient and other caregivers, is important in preventing the progression of complications that may lead to limb loss.

SIX

Aging and the Foot

This chapter will discuss common foot and ankle concerns for older adults and provide some tips on how to prevent or manage these concerns.

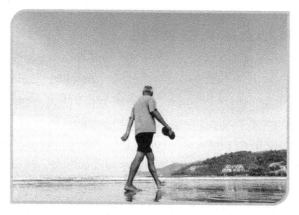

As many seniors know, the "golden years" can be very enriching—but they can also present challenges in the form of various aches and pains from foot and ankle conditions.

For older adults, foot and ankle problems can develop or worsen with age. These problems include deformities (such as bunions, flatfeet, and hammertoe), skin and nail changes, decreased bone strength, and arthritis. In addition, age often impacts other aspects of your health that can affect your feet. Let's take a look at each of these concerns.

FOOT DEFORMITIES

With age, deformities such as bunions, hammertoe, and flatfeet can become more problematic. Many of these conditions are progressive, which means they can become more pronounced over time. Not only can the symptoms get worse, but sometimes they can also cause pressure problems like corns and calluses. Also, as the foot ages, it can become stiffer, making it more difficult to get relief simply by using cushions, inserts, or pads.

SKIN AND NAIL CHANGES

Skin changes also occur with age, and these changes can bring on new problems in the feet. In older adults, the skin increasingly becomes thinner and frailer, sometimes resembling tissue paper. This can make the foot more susceptible to problems caused by rubbing and irritation, such as developing wounds, corns, and calluses. As already noted, deformities such as hammertoes can also lead to corns and calluses. In addition, the foot's natural cushioning, or footpads, become thinner with age, causing pain and aching when walking or standing.

AGE-RELATED TOENAIL CHANGES

Toenails also change as we age. In older people, toenails often become thickened or discolored, making it very difficult to trim them. Fungal infections affecting the toenails are also more common among seniors.

AGE-RELATED BONE CHANGES

The aging process can lead to weaker bones. As we age, it is not unusual for our bones to lose some of their density, which can result in osteoporosis, a common condition among older adults. For some seniors, lower bone density can be the cause of stress fractures in the foot. A stress fracture is a hairline break in the bone. Without treatment, a stress fracture can progress to a full fracture.

ARTHRITIS

Arthritis is a painful condition that can strike any joint in the body—often the joints in the knees, hips, hands, and feet. Osteoarthritis—the most common type of this disease— is associated with the "wear and tear" of the body, and it gets worse with age. This very common form of arthritis in older adults can occur in the big toe or in the ankle, making walking difficult.

OTHER HEALTH PROBLEMS

In addition to dealing with the previously mentioned foot and ankle problems, seniors are susceptible to other health concerns that can affect the feet. First, a person's general ability to heal tends to decrease with age, and that could slow down the recovery of foot problems. A second issue related to the aging process is high blood pressure, or hypertension, which is more likely to develop as someone gets older. Hypertension can lead to fluid retention and swelling in the feet and legs, which can make you more predisposed to developing sores—or ulcers—in the feet. A third concern is diabetes, which can develop at any age but often worsens as time goes on. Poor eyesight related to diabetes can make it difficult to care for your feet or detect sores. Diabetes can also produce nerve damage in the feet, creating a loss of sensation. And a fourth health concern that is more common in older people is gout, an extremely painful form of arthritis that often affects the big toe.

WHAT CAN YOU DO?

Now that we've reviewed the foot and ankle problems that many older people deal with, you may be wondering what you can do to protect your feet. Here are some guidelines based on the specific issue.

FOOT DEFORMITIES

Most deformities such as bunions, hammertoes, and flatfeet can't be prevented because they reflect particular biomechanics of the foot. However, effective treatments for these and other deformities are available by seeing a foot and ankle specialist. The specialist will carefully evaluate your feet and ankles and will create an appropriate treatment plan for you. Often, nonsurgical treatment options such as footwear modifications, padding, shoe inserts or custom orthotics, or corticosteroid injections will bring about effective pain relief. In some cases, however, surgery may be necessary to relieve the symptoms. Your foot and ankle specialist will determine whether surgery is appropriate for you.

SKIN PROBLEMS

What can you do to prevent or manage skin problems on your feet? Examining your feet, including looking carefully at the bottoms of your feet, is essential to make sure there are no cracks, cuts, or red spots that could indicate something is causing pressure on your foot.

CORNS AND CALLUSES

To help prevent cracks and cuts, keep your feet soft and moisturized. To help prevent corns and calluses, make sure your shoes fit properly. Also, as mentioned earlier, some calluses and corns are caused by other conditions, such as hammertoe or arthritis, so these problems should be addressed. Your foot and ankle specialist can shave down your corns or calluses using a surgical blade in the office. There are also measures you can take at home. You can apply a topical medicine to help keep a callus or corn from returning. Also, you can use an over-the-counter thin padding over the affected area to help reduce friction.

TOENAIL PROBLEMS

Toenail problems require the help of a foot and ankle specialist who can advise on proper footwear, treat any fungal infection that is present with medication, and properly trim the nails.

STRESS FRACTURES

To help reduce the likelihood of developing stress fractures, here are a few tips: Because stress fractures are often caused by overuse, be careful you don't overdo exercise; instead, build up to it gradually. Also, it's important that you wear supportive shoes and avoid walking on uneven surfaces. Since osteoporosis can be an underlying cause of stress fractures, be sure you're doing all you can for good bone health. Your doctor can advise you on steps to take to protect your bones, such as getting enough calcium and vitamin D. If you develop pain in your foot, be sure to see a foot and ankle specialist for an evaluation. This specialist will also advise you on appropriate activities and footwear. Possible treatments for stress fractures include rest, immobilization through a walking cast, or, in some cases, surgery.

ARTHRITIS

Arthritis can't be prevented, but there are strategies that can help reduce the pain. Activities should be modified so that they don't aggravate the arthritis. This is the focus of many fitness classes for seniors, which provide low-impact exercise and avoid incline work or repetitive stress or strain. With arthritis of the big toe, it's also important to minimize bending of that toe by wearing shoes with more rigid soles and by avoiding activity that involves toe work. For people with severe ankle arthritis, ankle replacement surgery is a possible option to eliminate the pain. In this procedure, similar to hip and knee replacement surgeries, the patient receives an implant that replaces the arthritic joint.

VISIT A FOOT SPECIALIST FOR ROUTINE FOOT CARE

You should make an appointment with a foot and ankle specialist to receive help with your routine foot care. As people get older, it often becomes difficult to handle the tasks needed to take care of our feet. Many seniors find it increasingly challenging to use instruments such as clippers and nail files. What's more, their eyesight can be a problem. This is why routine foot care is among the most common reasons that older adults visit a foot and ankle specialist. So if you think you could use help with trimming your toenails or taking care of corns and calluses, don't hesitate to seek professional care. In addition, other problems you may be experiencing can be addressed at that time.

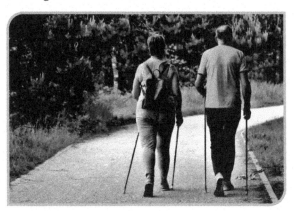

SEVEN

The Arthritic Foot

Arthritis is a medical term that describes inflammation of a joint. Joints are areas where two different bones contact one another. Some joints allow for motion to occur and some do not. The freedom of movement ranges from none (skull sutures) to fully mobile (hip, shoulder) with varying ranges in between. Each foot has thirty-three joints, all with different degrees of freedom of motion. With so many joints and with the strain that feet have to withstand, the feet are commonly affected by arthritis. There are two main types of arthritis that affect the human body: inflammatory arthritis and degenerative arthritis, also known as osteoarthritis. Examples of inflammatory arthritis are rheumatoid, psoriatic, gout, Lyme, ankylosing spondylitis, and septic arthritis.

 With inflammatory arthritis, something causes an immune response in the soft tissue surrounding the joint, called the joint capsule. If unchecked, the immune response can lead to weakening of the supportive structures around the joint, ligaments, and tendons, which can lead to instability, dislocation, and deformity. Inflammatory arthritis rarely damages the cartilage directly, but the inflammatory response can disrupt the synovial tissue, the main source of nutritional support, leading to secondary degeneration. Degenerative arthritis is caused by abnormal wear and tear of the cartilage, the smooth tissue that lines the ends of bones. Degenerative arthritis is a slow, progressive process, occurring over many years. Most joints in the body can show degenerative changes over time. Abnormal alignments or traumatic events involving a joint can lead to faster progression and earlier onset of degenerative changes.

Arthritis is diagnosed through a combination of medical history, physical examination, imaging studies, and laboratory testing. Clues to the type of arthritis can be found in the history of the condition (for example, time of onset, speed of progression, location 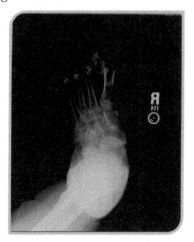 of symptoms, history of trauma, length of time stiffness, etc.) Physical examination reveals if there is a deformity, swelling, redness, increased temperature, or pain with palpation or motion. X-rays can identify deformities and provide radiographic clues to the type of arthritis, such as erosions, cysts, and joint space narrowing. Ultrasound, CT, and MRI tests may also be needed for a definitive diagnosis. Laboratory studies focus on identifying inflammatory and immune factors in the blood as well as changes in the white blood cell count. Joint fluid analysis can also be helpful for arriving at a diagnosis.

Nonsurgical treatment of arthritis focuses on three areas: inflammation reduction, joint support and stabilization, and strengthening surrounding musculature. Inflammation can be reduced with oral medications, injectable medications, topical medications, and physical therapy modalities. Usually some combination of the above is used. Certain arthritic conditions such as rheumatoid and psoriatic arthritis are considered autoimmune conditions and may need to be treated with immunosuppressive medications. Joint support and stability is achieved with various orthopedic appliances, ranging from taping to rigid bracing, based on individual needs. Strengthening of the supporting musculature is achieved by employing specific exercises, commonly directed by a physical therapist or other health professional.

The majority of arthritis patients I see in clinical practice as a podiatrist have degenerative arthritis. Any joint of the foot can be affected, but the big toe joint, ankle, and subtalar joints are the most commonly problematic. After arriving at the diagnosis and ruling out other issues, treatment

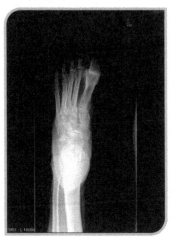

can be initiated. As mentioned before, degenerative arthritis commonly has a low-grade inflammatory component. Reducing this inflammation should be the first step in treatment.

An injection of anti-inflammatory medication directly into the involved joint is the fastest way to reduce joint inflammation. Fluoroscopy or ultrasound can be helpful for joint identification and needle guidance. A short series of two to three weekly injections is usually effective at reducing this inflammatory component. You can also use a combination therapy with oral and/or topical anti-inflammatories. CBD products, either orally ingested or topically applied, can also be helpful at reducing symptoms. Temporary immobilization of the affected joint using taping, bracing, or casting may be needed in some cases. Long-term stabilization of the foot joints is achieved using custom-molded foot orthotics. With ankle involvement, ankle-foot orthotics may be needed. Footwear is an important and commonly overlooked area to consider with arthritis patients. Areas to consider when selecting footwear for the arthritic patient are: accommodation of deformities, support and stability, and accommodation for orthotics and braces. Fortunately, there are a number of manufacturers that make a variety of shoes that are appropriate for the arthritis patient. Some good ones include Propét®, New Balance, Anodyne, Vionic®, and Dr. Comfort®. Professional sizing and fitting is important for a successful result.

Should symptoms persist after anti-inflammatory measures are used, physical therapy modalities can be employed. Class 4 laser therapy is a newer modality that is very effective at reducing pain and inflammation. Ten-to twenty-minute applications one to two times a week for three to four weeks is a typical protocol. Other modalities that can be used include ultrasound, electrical stimulation, hydrotherapy, paraffin, and infrared. Rehabilitation can begin after the inflammatory response is under control. Exercises prescribed are based on the joints involved and other patient-specific needs. You may need a consultation with a physiatrist or physical therapist. Inflammatory arthritis is treated in a similar manner. Input from the patient's primary care doctor and rheumatologist should be sought for managing their medications, particularly for those on immunosuppressants. Anyone with persistent joint pain in their feet and legs should have an evaluation by a foot and ankle specialist right away. Like most medical conditions, early intervention is important to protect and preserve joint structure and function.

EIGHT

Bunions

The bunion deformity, technically termed hallux abductovalgus (HAV), is much more than just a bump of bone growing on the foot. It is a three-dimensional positional misalignment of the entire first ray of the foot, which includes the big toe and the first metatarsal. Ill-fitting shoes do not cause bunions, although the wrong shoes can make a bunion more painful. Bunions are usually hereditary and can appear at any age, but most people begin to notice them in their later teen years. Other causes of bunions are certain traumas and arthritic conditions that disrupt the normal anatomic stabilizing structures.

It is thought by most biomechanical experts that bunions are caused by an unstable first ray. This first-ray instability is often related to rearfoot joint instability, particularly in the subtalar and midtarsal joint complex. Rearfoot instability allows the talus bone to slide out of position and move forward, downward, and medially. This leads to an excessively pronated position of the foot. In this position,

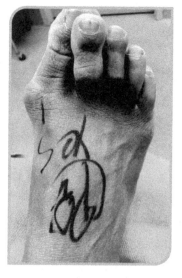

the arch appears to flatten as the foot rolls inward. If this pronated position persists during the gait cycle when the foot should be returning to the more stable supinated position, then the mechanical effectiveness of the main muscular stabilizer of the first ray (the peroneus longus) is effectively reduced. This relative weakness combined with inherited joint surface changes and ligament laxity allows for three-plane first-ray instability. The first ray should be stabilized against the ground to prepare the foot for toe off. With first-ray instability, the first ray gets pushed upward by the force of body weight, making it raised or elevated relative to the other metatarsals. This can allow the foot to pronate even more, compounding the rearfoot instability. With continued stress, the first ray will begin to twist into a position of valgus. This position can be visualized in the extreme with the toenail of the big toe no longer facing straight up but rather facing the other foot. The first metatarsal will begin to move away from the midline of the foot and protrude on the medial or inside of the foot. Most bunion symptoms begin with this bony prominence interacting with footwear. With progression of the deformity, severe joint misalignment can occur, leading to joint damage and arthritis. Bunions progress at different rates for different people. Like most conditions, early intervention can prevent later problems.

CONSERVATIVE CARE

Although we cannot say that bunions can be prevented, it is my belief from twenty-five years of treating this condition that controlling abnormal foot mechanics can not only reduce the symptoms of a bunion but also slow down or even halt its progression.

Abnormal mechanics can be controlled with orthopedic devices such as foot orthotics and braces. One of the most effective ways to address foot mechanical issues is with custom-molded foot orthotics. These devices are made specifically to the shape of a person's foot by taking a cast, foam impression, or scan to capture an accurate shape. Corrections are then added to the devices based on the biomechanical findings of the foot and ankle specialist. These devices fit in most shoes and can be moved between shoes. Off-the-shelf devices tend to be less effective at controlling foot mechanics due to their materials and lack of corrective changes based on patient examination. Extreme levels of instability may require bracing that extends above the ankle, known as an ankle-foot orthotic (AFO). These are also custom constructed based on a mold of the foot and leg.

Many devices have been designed to attempt to realign the bunion deformity without surgery. Although some may provide a measure of symptom relief, I have yet to find any to be effective in changing the position of the toe on a long-term basis. As noted, conservative care for bunions focuses on preventing symptoms and ensuring rearfoot stability. Accommodation of the bunion bump and toe angulation during shoe wearing is the next step.

Shoes should be wide enough to accommodate the bony prominence. Trace the shape of the foot with a pencil and paper and measure the width at the bunion area. Having stretchable materials such as Lycra® in the upper area of the shoe can be helpful in reducing pressure on the bump. Custom-molded orthopedic shoes are another option if conventional or extra-depth shoes don't offer comfort. There are many padding options available, including foam, gels, rubber, felt, lambswool, and cotton, in various shapes and sizes. A foot and ankle specialist or pedorthist (footwear expert) can help with these accommodations.

As with many foot and ankle conditions, abnormal mechanics are the root of the problem. A thorough examination by a foot and ankle specialist is the best way to get the right recommendations for your particular set of circumstances.

Should surgery be needed, be sure to get more than one opinion from a board-certified foot and ankle surgeon who is well versed in bunion correction.

SURGICAL CARE

If you should look into surgical options, there are many. Because bunions stem from a hypermobile rearfoot, options range from minimally invasive joint stabilization to major bone reconstructions and joint fusions. I favor minimally invasive stabilization procedures whenever possible, such as the extra-osseous talotarsal stabilization procedure that uses a titanium implant. This technique allows for a relatively short weight-bearing recovery versus a lengthy immobilization and weight-bearing restrictions that other bone procedures require. Once rearfoot stability is ensured with orthotics or surgery, the bunion deformity can be addressed.

BUNION SURGERY OPTIONS

As mentioned above, a bunion is a positional that can lead to pain with shoe wearing and walking. Conservative treatment is always favored; however, the only way to truly eliminate the deformity itself is by surgical correction. Bunion surgery has been performed for over 100 years, with many procedures and variations known. Advances in bone-fixation techniques have improved the outcomes and longevity of bunion correction surgery over the last thirty years. There are three main surgical approaches to non-arthritic bunion deformity.

NON-ARTHRITIC BUNION OPTIONS

SIMPLE BUNIONECTOMY

In this procedure, the bunion "bump" is reduced or removed with various surgical instruments. This type of procedure has the shortest average recovery time and lends itself to minimally invasive techniques. It does not, however, address the three-plane nature of the deformity and the associated soft-tissue imbalances that occur in the HAV deformity, thus making recurrence of the condition likely over time. Adding soft-tissue release–rebalancing and/or adductor tendon transposition can help address the underlying issues and lessen the recurrence rates. The typical recovery time is three to four weeks in a surgical shoe, followed by three to four weeks in sneakers or other roomy footwear. Impact activities can usually resume after four weeks as tolerated. My preference is to reserve this type of procedure for mild deformities or for patients whose bone quality would make bone procedures ill-advised.

FIRST METATARSAL OSTEOTOMY

In this procedure, the first metatarsal bone is cut and repositioned to reduce the deformity. This type of procedure has numerous techniques. The most commonly performed is the distal chevron osteotomy, also known as the Austin bunionectomy. A small surgical saw is used to cut through the metatarsal at the end closest to the toe. The end of the bone is then shifted toward the second metatarsal and secured to the other segment with a small screw or pin for stability during bone healing. The geometry of the bone cut makes it very stable, allowing for immediate postoperative protected weight-bearing. It is also not a three-plane correction. As with the simple bunionectomy, adding soft-tissue release–rebalancing and tendon transposition can help improve the correction and reduce recurrence rates. This is a versatile procedure that can address the mild to moderate bunion effectively. It has the advantage of being able to be performed in an office surgical suite setting under local anesthesia, potentially saving out-of-pocket costs for patients with high-deductible health plans. The recovery period is typically four to six weeks in a surgical shoe followed by four to six weeks in sneakers or other loose-fitting shoes. Impact activities can usually be resumed at eight to ten weeks.

LAPIDUS PROCEDURE

The Lapidus procedure is the only bunion correction that allows for a three-plane correction of all the components of the bunion deformity while also stabilizing the mechanical instability that caused the bunion to begin with. This 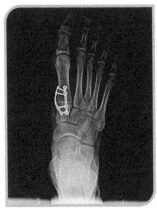 procedure involves fusing the joint between the first metatarsal and the bone behind it, the medial cuneiform bone. Advances in instrumentation and fixation allow for precise correction and strong fixation, thus enabling immediate protected weight-bearing in a CAM walking boot. Protected weight-bearing in the boot must last for six to eight weeks followed by sneakers or other roomy shoes for an additional four to six weeks. Impact activities can usually resume after three months. Recurrence rates for this procedure are extremely low due to the complete three-plane correction and the stability of the fusion procedure.

ARTHRITIC BUNION OPTIONS

Some bunion deformities are related to arthritic conditions: rheumatoid arthritis, gout, post-traumatic arthritis, and others. In addition, a long-standing bunion deformity can cause premature wear of the joint surfaces, which then leads to degenerative arthritis. When arthritis is present in the big toe joint, the previously described approaches to the condition can improve the appearance of the bunion but may result in a painful, stiff joint if the arthritis is not addressed. The arthritic bunion deformity requires a different approach. There are also three main ways to address an arthritic bunion.

ARTHROPLASTY

Arthroplasty of the big toe joint, also called the Keller procedure, is the simplest of the three approaches. This involves removing part of the joint along with the bunion bump. Usually, soft tissue from around the joint is placed in the space where the bone was removed to act as a spacer. This procedure has a similar recovery to a simple bunionectomy. Motion of the toe joint remains after surgery, but some loss of strength of toe flexion is typical. This procedure works well for mild to moderate deformities. Larger deformities may have a tendency for recurrence due to the instability of the toe from joint removal.

IMPLANT ARTHROPLASTY

Implant arthroplasty involves removing the entire joint and replacing it with artificial components. Many materials have been used for big toe joint replacement. The best type of device for the arthritic bunion condition is the semi-constrained silastic implant. These devices can hold the big toe in a corrected position after surgery, making them useful with larger deformities. The main drawback with implants is the fact that the materials do not last forever. Materials and/or the bone surrounding the implant can degenerate over time, leading to implant failure and the need for revision. The usual life span of most artificial joints is ten to fifteen years. Recovery time from implant arthroplasty is similar to a first metatarsal osteotomy procedure.

ARTHRODESIS

Arthrodesis of the big toe joint is the only permanent solution to the arthritic bunion deformity. It can also provide three-plane correction and stability of the first ray, making it useful for larger deformities. Advanced fixation techniques allow for immediate protected weight-bearing in a CAM walking boot. Recovery time is similar to the Lapidus procedure. The functionality of the fused big toe joint is actually very good. It has even been performed successfully in high-level athletes. The biggest problem with the fused big toe joint is that it limits the ability to wear higher heeled shoes.

METATARSUS ADDUCTUS

Up to 30 percent of bunion patients also have the condition metatarsus adductus, where all of the metatarsal bones angle toward the midline of the body. Significant metatarsus adductus prevents accurate three-plane correction of the bunion deformity. In these cases, the adjacent metatarsals 2 and 3 may need to be straightened first to allow first-ray correction. These procedures can be performed during the same surgical session through a separate incision.

HOW TO CHOOSE THE BEST PROCEDURE FOR YOU

Start with a consultation with a board-certified foot and ankle specialist. They will do a comprehensive evaluation and review of imaging studies. When deciding on a surgical approach, multiple factors should be considered and the plan should be individualized for each patient. Seek a second opinion if you are unsure of what direction to take. Surgical management should only be considered after carefully weighing your options and the benefits and risks of all approaches.

Nine

Metatarsal Problems

METATARSALGIA

Metatarsalgia is the term for pain in the metatarsal area. There are several structures that can become painful in the metatarsal area including the skin, soft tissue, tendons, ligaments, joints, and nerves. It is often hard to pinpoint if there was a trauma before the onset of pain. Occasionally traumatic events, such as stepping on a hard object barefoot, can be the cause of injury to this area. Most often, chronic overload of the forefoot area due to mechanical imbalances leads to increased tissue stress, which leads to injury and inflammation. For treatment, your doctor needs an accurate determination of which structures are injured and a diagnosis of contributing mechanical imbalances and/or shoe gear factors that have led to the injury. Physical examination of the area can help pinpoint structures involved. Imaging studies such as x-rays, ultrasounds, and MRIs can also be used to arrive at a diagnosis. Biomechanical examination of the joints of the lower extremities and shoe gear evaluation can help determine contributing factors. Treatment begins with reducing the inflammation in the area and temporarily off-loading the area to reduce tissue stress. Oral anti-inflammatories, physical therapy modalities, and cortisone injections may be employed for inflammation reduction. Stretching exercises especially for the posterior foot and leg muscles are important for reducing forefoot strain at push off. Correcting mechanical imbalances with foot orthotics or braces is necessary to allow the tissues to recover fully and prevent recurrence of inflammation. Surgical intervention for metatarsalgia is uncommon and usually involves shortening or elevating a prominent metatarsal.

MORTON'S NEUROMA

Morton's neuroma is a nerve condition of the common digital nerve that starts between two metatarsals and branches into two of the toes. The most commonly affected nerve is between the third and fourth metatarsals. This condition is not a true nerve tumor as the name suggests. It usually begins as inflammation around the nerve. After prolonged periods without treatment, scar tissue can develop around the nerve, which resembles a tumor on visual inspection. When the nerve is enlarged, it can be felt clicking between the metatarsals during a physical exam. A diagnostic ultrasound can help confirm the diagnosis and measure the thickness of the nerve. An MRI can be used as well, especially when ruling out other causes of pain in the area.

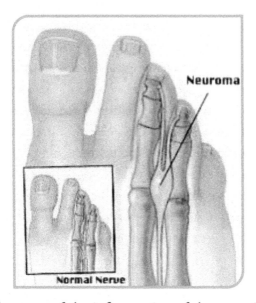

Neuroma

Normal Nerve

The cause of the inflammation of the nerve is most often chronic trauma to the area that presses the nerve against the ligament that holds the two metatarsals together. Biomechanical imbalances that lead to rearfoot and forefoot instability are usually the cause of the mechanical overload of the forefoot. Treatment is similar to that for metatarsalgia— inflammation reduction followed by mechanical stabilization with foot orthotics. An ultrasound-guided cortisone injection to the area of the inflamed nerve is an effective way to reduce inflammation rapidly. A small series of one to three injections one to two weeks apart will usually resolve the acute symptoms. Mechanical control of any contributing imbalances is necessary to allow the nerve to recover fully and prevent recurrent trauma.

Sometimes, the damage to the nerve may be permanent. In these cases, symptoms will persist despite treatment and mechanical control. Chemoneurolysis is a technique that can be used to treat chronic neuroma pain. This technique involves injecting the affected nerve with 4 percent ethanol solution in a series of three to seven weekly injections. Although we don't know these injections' exact mechanism of action, they tend to permanently block the pain fibers of the nerve that runs along the outside of the nerve sheath. Sensory fibers tend to not be affected by these injections. On rare occasions, neuromas can be resistant to all conservative treatment. In these cases, surgical removal of the affected neuroma will relieve the pain. A small area of residual numbness between the toes does result, but most people don't notice this after a while.

SESAMOIDITIS

The big toe-joint complex has two small accessory bones that reside beneath the first metatarsal head and are within the short flexor tendon and joint lining. The function of these bones is akin to our kneecap; they increase the mechanical advantage of the short flexor tendon, which stabilizes the big toe against the ground during the push-off phase of walking. Inflammation in the area of the sesamoid bones is called sesamoiditis. Inflammation is usually the result of trauma to the area. Acute trauma, such as stepping on a hard object or forcefully bending the toe upward, can result in inflammation to the area. Chronic overload to the area such as with a plantarflexed first metatarsal, cavus foot, or hallux hammertoe can also result in inflammation of the sesamoid area.

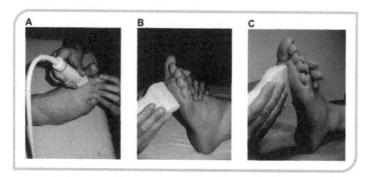

With a bunion deformity, the sesamoid bones can get out of alignment, which can cause increased pressure and stress, resulting in inflammation to the area. X-rays can help to rule out fractures or other bone abnormalities. A diagnostic ultrasound is helpful in localizing the inflammation and ruling out injuries to the tendons and ligaments in the area.

Treatment of sesamoiditis includes reducing inflammation and pressure to the area. Inflammation can be reduced with oral anti-inflammatories, physical medicine, modalities, or cortisone injections to the area. Off-loading with a dancer's pad can relieve stress on the area temporarily. Custom foot orthotics with a dancer's pad modification can provide long-term pressure relief. Acute fractures and stress fractures of the sesamoid bones can be a source of pain in this area. These are treated with off-loading as with sesamoiditis and physical therapy modalities to reduce pain and swelling. Delayed healing of these fractures can be treated with electromagnetic or ultrasound bone stimulators.

Surgical management can be considered in cases that don't respond to conservative care. Options include correcting the underlying structural abnormalities like hammertoe, bunion, plantar-flexed metatarsal, or cavus foot. Removal of a chronically inflamed sesamoid can also be considered. Displaced acute fractures of a sesamoid can be treated with surgical reduction and fixation. Unresponsive non-unions can be surgically treated with bone grafting or removal of the fractured sesamoid.

TEN

Foot and Ankle Trauma

Injuries to the foot and ankle are common. Many injuries are caused by chronic, repetitive trauma over time. This chapter will focus on acute injuries to the foot and ankle that I commonly see in clinical practice.

LACERATIONS

A laceration is a cut or tear in the skin. These are typically caused by sharp objects such as glass or metal. Lacerations most often occur on the bottom of the foot from stepping on a sharp object. They can occur on the top of the foot as well from dropping a sharp object on the foot or kicking something sharp. Laceration treatment varies based on the severity of the injury and degree of contamination. Minor lacerations can be treated with cleansing and local wound care. More severe lacerations should be thoroughly irrigated and inspected for foreign material and injury to deeper structures. If a laceration is clean and less than twenty-four hours old, it can be closed with adhesive strips or sutures. Older injuries need to be left open to heal from the inside out. Severely contaminated wounds need to be washed out with a pulsed pressurized solution in an operating room setting. A tetanus shot should be considered for those who haven't had a booster in more than ten years. Antibiotic treatment can be topical for clean wounds. Contaminated wounds require oral antibiotics to prevent infection.

FOREIGN BODIES

The most common foreign bodies that get lodged in the foot are wood splinters and glass fragments.

Most penetrating foreign bodies occur on the bottom of the feet. Often, these can be removed in the office without any need for anesthesia. Foreign bodies that are deeper may need to be removed under local anesthetic. Sometimes, a small incision must be made to get the foreign bodies. Occasionally, foreign bodies can be driven deep into the foot, well below the skin. In many instances, these can be left in place. If they are small enough, our bodies will grow tissue around the object to wall it off. Should they remain symptomatic or act as a source of infection, operative exploration under regional or general anesthesia may be needed. MRI studies can be helpful to locate deep foreign bodies and assist with planning for removal.

NAIL AVULSION

Traumatic nail avulsion (a nail pulled off the nail bed) usually occurs from striking the toe against a hard object.

My treatment preference is to convert partial nail avulsions to complete to fully evaluate the nail bed for damage and allow for adequate wound care. The nail bed has a lot of blood vessels, so these injuries can bleed a lot, but the bleeding can usually be controlled with pressure and elevation. In some cases, topical medications may be needed to stop the bleeding. Underlying nail bed lacerations should be repaired with sutures. Wound care should be performed daily using nonadhesive dressings until the nail bed skin heals over. The new nail will begin to grow within a few weeks and can take six months or more to grow in completely.

SUBUNGUAL HEMATOMA

Subungual hematoma refers to a collection of blood or tissue fluid under a toenail. This can be the result of sudden trauma to the toe like kicking a hard object or having the toe stepped on, or chronic trauma such as wearing the wrong sized footwear for an extended period. Pain comes from the pressure of the fluid on the underlying nail bed since the nail itself cannot expand. Prompt pain relief is attained by draining the fluid from beneath the nail. This can often be performed without anesthesia by inserting a sterile needle under the far edge of the nail. Once drained, a dressing is maintained for a few days to collect any additional fluid drainage. Most often, a new nail will form under the current nail plate. A new nail will take at least six months to grow. At some point, the old nail will become loose and fall off, revealing the new nail underneath. A partially loosened nail can be secured with tape to prevent it from being snagged in socks or shoes and being forcefully torn off.

TOE SPRAIN

Blunt trauma to one or more of the toes can result in injury to the joint-supporting structures or to the bones. A sprain is an injury to the ligaments around the joints. Sprains are treated with temporary immobilization by splinting the toe to the neighboring toe. This is called a buddy splint. Rest, ice, and elevation are prescribed for the first week to reduce pain and swelling. Splinting should be maintained for two to four weeks to allow the ligaments to heal. If the injury is to the metatarsal joint, the foot can be placed in a surgical shoe for the two- to four-week period for protection.

TOE DISLOCATION

A dislocation means that the joint injury resulted in the joint being out of alignment. Dislocations require reduction (putting the joint back in alignment). This can usually be done without a surgical incision under local anesthesia. The toe can then be treated with splintage for four to six weeks. Occasionally, stability cannot be maintained with a splint alone. In these cases, a metal pin can be inserted through the toe after reduction to maintain alignment while healing. The pin is then removed after four to six weeks.

TOE FRACTURE

A fracture is a break in one of the toe bones. If the fracture fragments are well aligned and minimally separated, treatment can be similar to a toe sprain: using a splint. For fractures, splintage should be maintained until signs of healing show up on an x-ray. This is usually four to six weeks. Displaced or malaligned fractures should be reduced similarly to dislocations. Fractures that cannot be properly reduced without surgery may need surgical reduction and stabilization.

TURF TOE

Turf toe is a term used for an injury to the ligaments around the big toe joint. Often, the mechanism of injury is the forceful bending of the foot when the front part is stuck to the ground. This was a common injury on earlier versions of artificial turf surfaces, hence the name. The severity of this injury can range from mild sprains to partial or complete dislocations. Temporary immobilization with a stiff-soled shoe to prevent toe bending is needed in most cases. Dislocations and associated displaced fractures would require reduction prior to immobilization. More severe injuries require a period of non-weight-bearing using crutches or a knee scooter.

METATARSAL FRACTURES

The metatarsal bones are the bones just behind each toe. There are five, with the first metatarsal being the thickest and strongest. Metatarsal fractures can occur from direct trauma, such as dropping a heavy object on the foot, or indirect trauma, such as twisting the foot forcefully. Non-displaced fractures can be treated with immobilization in a walking boot until an x-ray shows signs of healing, typically six to eight weeks. Displaced fractures and those that involve joint surfaces usually require surgical reduction and stabilization. A

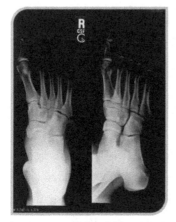

period of non-weight-bearing is usually required following surgical reduction, followed by walking boot weight-bearing for six to eight weeks. One kind of metatarsal fracture that almost always requires surgical intervention, whether displaced or not, is the Jones fracture. This fracture occurs in a part of the fifth metatarsal, where the blood supply is poor. This makes these fractures notoriously hard to heal. Most of the medical literature suggests surgical repair for reduced healing time and improved functional outcome.

LISFRANC JOINT INJURY

A Lisfranc joint injury is one that we don't hear about regularly. It certainly has an unusual name. The Lisfranc joint is where the five metatarsal bones connect to the rest of the foot. It is roughly in the middle of the foot. This joint is named after a French surgeon from the 1800s who described injuries to this area happening to cavalry soldiers who fell from horses with their feet caught in the stirrups. Unfortunately, the only treatment at the time was amputation of the front part of the foot. Fortunately, we have better options now!

The Lisfranc joint is a very stable joint that contributes to the structure of the arch. The many ligaments and bone interlocking also contribute to the stability of this joint. Injury to this complex requires a significant force. Automobile or motorcycle accidents and falls from heights are the most common causes of this injury. It can be caused in sports when a force is applied above the foot, such as a tackler, while the front part of the foot is stuck to the playing surface. This causes tearing of one or more of the ligaments stabilizing the joint. Occasionally, fractures of the bones in the area can occur as well.

A high index of suspicion is needed in diagnosing these injuries, as x-ray findings can be subtle or absent. In some cases, stress x-rays, during which force is applied to attempt to move the joint, may be necessary to perform under anesthesia to arrive at the diagnosis. Mild cases without fracture or displacement can usually be managed with a period of non-weight-bearing immobilization for four to six weeks followed by rehabilitation. Cases with displacement, fractures, or gross instability need surgical intervention. Surgical options include closed reduction with percutaneous pinning and open reduction with internal fixation. The choice of procedure is based on the severity of the injury, the injury pattern, and the reducibility of the injury. A period of non-weight-bearing for six to eight weeks is needed. Non-weight-bearing rehab exercises can start as soon as swelling and pain have reduced after surgery. Surgical hardware is commonly removed after healing. Full recovery can take six months or more.

REARFOOT FRACTURES

Traumatic fractures of the rearfoot bones usually occur through high-energy mechanisms such as a fall from a height or a motor vehicle accident. Treatment of these fractures is based on the severity of injury, displacement, joint involvement, soft-tissue integrity, and patient health. Nonsurgical and surgical methods can be used depending on the above factors. Almost all rearfoot fractures require prolonged non-weight-bearing for proper healing. Two to three months of non-weight-bearing followed by using a walking boot for an additional two to three months is typical.

ANKLE SPRAINS

Injury to the ligaments around the ankle joint are usually caused by twisting type of movements during sports or with a fall. There are ligaments on the inside and outside of the ankle joint. The outside, or lateral, ligaments are the most commonly injured. There are three distinct ligaments on the lateral, or outer, side of the ankle. The most commonly injured one is just in front of the outside anklebone, the fibula. This ligament attaches the fibula to the talus foot bone. The second most commonly injured ligament is just below the tip of the fibula bone. This ligament attaches the fibula to the heel bone. The third lateral ligament is behind the fibula and also attaches to the talus foot bone. This ligament is rarely injured in an ankle sprain. Most sprains affect the anterior talofibular ligament and the calcaneofibular ligament to varying degrees. Most sprains of the ankle can be treated with temporary immobilization in a laced ankle brace with rehabilitation starting after one to two weeks. Should there be instability of the joint, cast immobilization and non-weight-bearing may be needed for an initial four weeks prior to active rehabilitation. Surgical treatment is rarely needed for acute ankle sprains. However, some patients may develop chronic instability after injury, especially with a history of multiple sprains. These patients may benefit from surgical ligament reconstruction.

ANKLE FRACTURES

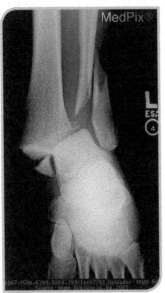

Fracture of the anklebones can follow the same mechanisms that cause ankle sprains but with greater energy. They can also result from falls or motor vehicle accidents. Either or both of the anklebones, the tibia and fibula, can break in one or more places. Treatment is based on severity, displacement, joint involvement, soft-tissue integrity, and patient health. Nonsurgical and surgical methods may be employed. Anatomic alignment of the joint surfaces is the ideal goal to reduce the likelihood of post-traumatic arthritis in the future. A period of non-weight-bearing immobilization is needed, depending on fracture type, severity, treatment, etc. Rehabilitation can start earlier after surgical repair due to the stability of the fixation hardware. This can help the injured person return to activity faster.

TENDON INJURIES

Tendons are soft-tissue structures that connect muscles to bones and enable us to move a body part. Tendon trauma in the foot and ankle can occur by a penetrating injury or laceration as well as by indirect trauma such as a rapid positional change. Injuries to tendons vary in severity from inflammation to partial tearing to complete rupture. There are more than two dozen tendons in each foot. The most commonly injured tendons are the extensor and flexor tendons of the big toe, the anterior tibial tendon, the posterior tibial tendon, the peroneal tendons, and the Achilles tendon. Doctors assess the severity of tendon injury through examination as with ultrasound and MRI imaging modalities. Minor injuries to tendons result in an inflammation called tendonitis. These injuries can be treated similarly to sprains, with initial relative rest, ice, and elevation followed by rehabilitation exercises. Partial tendon tears are treated with temporary immobilization for four to six weeks to allow for healing and prevent complete rupture. Ice and elevation are also part of standard treatment. Mobilization exercises can begin once the acute inflammation subsides, followed by strengthening exercises and balance training. Complete tendon tears can be treated similarly, provided the two ends of the tendon are close to one another. Rigid immobilization in a cast is needed to keep the ends close together while healing. If there is a significant distance between the torn ends of the tendon, surgical repair is needed. Surgical repair is followed by cast immobilization for four weeks followed by a rehabilitation program.

ELEVEN

Sports-Related Conditions of the Foot and Ankle

Many sports activities involve the foot and ankle, making them subject to overuse and injury. Sports medicine is a vast subject with full textbooks dedicated to the subject. This chapter will outline the most common sports-related conditions. However, acute injuries such as fractures, sprains, and tendon injuries were addressed in Chapter 10. This chapter will focus on the more chronic issues that typically result from repetitive trauma and/or mechanical imbalances.

BLACK TOENAILS

A black toenail is a result of blood beneath the nail that has dried. This can range from small spots under the nail to complete nail discoloration. Unlike the acute subungual hematoma (blood under the toenail), this condition is usually painless. It is caused by repetitive trauma to the toe box of footwear. This condition will resolve without treatment as nail growth replaces the discolored area of the nail. Sometimes, an entire new nail will form under the injured nail. In this case, the old nail will come off on its own as it is pushed off by the new nail growth. But be aware that injured toenails can lose the natural barrier to invasion by microorganisms. Chronic nail injury is a common precursor to nail fungal infections. Good foot hygiene and topical antifungal application can help prevent infection as the nail unit recovers.

METATARSAL STRESS FRACTURES

Stress fractures of the metatarsals occur from chronic, repetitive weight-bearing trauma. This injury was originally termed a march fracture because it was first diagnosed in military recruits who were forced to march long distances. This is a common injury in distance runners, but it can occur from any chronic overloading activity. Symptoms of a stress fracture usually come on gradually. The typical area of pain is near the base of one of the metatarsals in the middle of the foot. Pain is relieved with rest but returns with more weight-bearing activity. Stress injuries to a bone can range from inflammation within the bone to partial fracture to complete fracture with displacement.

A high index of suspicion is needed for diagnosis. Initial x-rays often show no signs of a fracture. Often, advanced imaging techniques like an MRI or a bone scan are necessary for a definitive diagnosis. Like any injury, treatment is guided by the severity. In the early stages of a stress injury, a reduction in training volume and/or intensity may be all that is needed to allow the bone to recover. More often, a period of restriction from the causative activity is needed. A break of four to six weeks is usually recommended with a gradual return to previous training volume and intensity after that. Non-weight-bearing cross training activities can be used to keep the athlete's fitness level up during recovery. Should pain be present with regular daily activities, protected weight-bearing in a surgical shoe or walking boot may be needed to protect the healing bone.

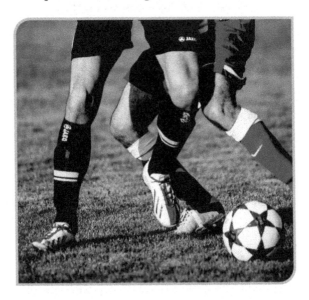

The goal of this early diagnosis and treatment is to prevent the stress fracture from progressing to a complete fracture, which can become displaced and malaligned. Displaced or malaligned metatarsal fractures or non-displaced fractures that fail to heal may require surgical intervention. Surgical reduction can be performed using local or regional anesthesia and usually includes some form of implant to stabilize the fracture following reduction. Non-weight-bearing immobilization for four to six weeks followed by a gradual return to weight-bearing is required after surgery. An alternative to surgery for nonhealing fractures is to use an electronic bone stimulator. These devices use either pulsed electromagnetic or pulsed ultrasound waves to stimulate healing and bone formation in a fracture.

TARSAL BONE STRESS FRACTURES

The tarsal bones are all of the other bones in the foot other than the toes and metatarsals. Stress fractures of the tarsal bones are rare due to the abundant blood supply in these bones. The most common tarsal stress fracture in sports occurs in the navicular bone, which is located in the middle of the foot just forward from the ankle. Stress fractures of the navicular are more common in high-impact sports such as gymnastics, figure skating, and martial arts, but they can occur in any weight-bearing activity. A usual sign is pain in the area of the navicular bone after activity that is slow to improve with rest. As with metatarsal stress fractures, tarsal bone fractures can be hard to see on initial x-rays. A CT scan, bone scan, or MRI is often needed for a definitive diagnosis.

Much of the medical literature recommends avoiding weight-bearing for treatment of tarsal stress fractures. I prefer protected weight-bearing in a walking boot, provided there is no fracture displacement or joint involvement. Recent research supports the notion that the stress of weight-bearing on a stable fracture can stimulate bone healing through bone callus formation. The usual protocol is four to six weeks of protected weight-bearing followed by a gradual return to activity. Fractures that fail to heal after appropriate treatment can be considered for bone stimulator use. Surgery can be considered for slow or nonhealing navicular fractures, such as displacement of tarsal stress fractures, which is a rare complication. Pins or screws can be placed through the skin using fluoroscopic x-rays for guidance. Established nonhealing fractures may need an open reduction with bone graft use. Stress fractures of the calcaneus or heel bone are the second most common tarsal stress fracture. These are usually caused by repetitive trauma, but they are difficult to see on plain x-rays. A bone scan or MRI may be needed to identify these injuries.

It is rare for calcaneal stress fractures to break through the outside of the bone and become complete fractures. Protected weight-bearing is used to allow the bone to heal. The heel bone has the best blood supply of all of the foot bones, so stress fractures heal readily. Often, all that is needed is a plastic heel cup to reduce shock through the bone during walking to allow the bone to heal. Walking boots can be considered for those who still have pain while using the heel cup only. Four to six weeks of protected weight-bearing followed by a gradual return to activity is the typical protocol.

TENDONITIS

There are over two dozen tendons in each foot. Any of the tendons of the foot can be subject to overloading and subsequent injury from sports. Subacute or chronic tendon injury usually results in inflammation of the tendon tissue, called tendonitis, or of the tissue surrounding certain tendons, termed tenosynovitis. The following are some of the more common tendon issues.

FLEXOR HALLUCIS LONGUS TENDONITIS

The flexor hallucis longus tendon stabilizes the big toe against the ground during walking. Injury to it can occur in activities where the big toe is bent upward repetitively, such as dancing or jumping. The most common locations for pain to occur with inflammation of this tendon are beneath the big toe joint. Here, the tendon runs through a narrow fibrous tunnel between two small bones called the sesamoid bones. Putting finger pressure between the two sesamoid bones will elicit pain. The pain often extends farther up the foot a few centimeters, which can help differentiate this condition from sesamoiditis, inflammation of the sesamoid apparatus itself.

A diagnostic ultrasound can be helpful in identifying which structures are involved. An ultrasound-guided injection of a soluble corticosteroid mixed with a local anesthetic into the tendon area can be of diagnostic and therapeutic value. Relative rest for two to four weeks followed by active rehabilitation will allow the inflammation to subside.

In ballet dancers who dance on their toes, the flexor hallucis longus can become inflamed in the back of the ankle. The inflamed tendon structures can become entrapped in the fibrous sheath that the tendon runs in, leading to triggering of the big toe. Triggering is when a digit gets stuck in a position with attempted motion. Rest from toe dancing for four weeks should allow for reduction of inflammation. A cortisone injection into the area of entrapment can be helpful for those who don't respond to rest.

EXTENSOR TENDONITIS

The extensor tendons run under the skin on the top of the foot and move the toes upward. Inflammation of the tendons or their sheaths can occur from direct pressure from footwear or from overuse, such as uphill running. Rest from the offending activity for two to three weeks usually helps. Footwear modification to avoid pressure on the top of the foot is usually necessary. A cortisone injection can be used in cases resistant to rest.

PERONEAL TENDONITIS

The peroneal tendons run along the outside of the ankle and foot. They can be injured during inversion-type ankle sprains. A high-arch foot type can put extra strain on the peroneal tendons, resulting in injury. Lack of adequate ankle bending during walking and running can cause an overuse of the peroneus brevis tendon due to compensatory outward turning of the foot to increase ankle motion. Pain is usually experienced on the outside of the ankle and foot. Rest and anti-inflammatory measures followed by active rehabilitation is the usual protocol. Again, a cortisone injection can be employed in cases resistant to rest. Occasionally, small tears between the fibers of the tendon can occur. These require longer periods of rest with immobilization in a walking boot, typically for four to six weeks. Surgical repair may be needed in large tears or ones that do not respond to immobilization.

POSTERIOR TIBIAL TENDONITIS

The posterior tibial tendon is on the inside of the ankle and foot. It is a major supporter of the arch of the foot. People with low-arch types or whose feet pronate, or roll inward, excessively can experience overuse injury to this tendon as it works to stabilize the arch against the abnormal forces. The most common area to feel pain from this condition is on the side of the foot at the peak of the arch. This is the main area where the tendon attaches to the bone. A similar protocol of rest and anti-inflammatory measures followed by active rehabilitation is employed. A cortisone injection can be used for resistant cases. Controlling abnormal foot mechanics with an orthotic arch support is usually necessary to help the tendon recover and to prevent recurrence.

ACHILLES TENDONITIS

The Achilles tendon is located at the back of the leg and attaches to the back of the heel bone. This tendon is the most commonly injured in sports. Injuries can run from mild inflammation to complete rupture. The two areas of the Achilles tendon where injuries occur are where it attaches to the heel bone and in the central area of the tendon. The central area of the tendon has the least amount of blood supply, making injuries to this area harder to heal. This is the area of the tendon where most Achilles tendon ruptures occur. Injuries to the central area of the tendon are therefore more serious and need to be treated aggressively.

Injuries to both areas will require a period of rest. Temporary immobilization may be needed and can range from taping to a walking boot. Heel lifts can be employed to reduce stress on the tendon. Physical therapy modalities such as laser and ultrasound can be used to reduce inflammation. Stretching and strength training can begin once pain has reduced. Oral anti-inflammatories can help to reduce inflammation. A cortisone injection in the Achilles tendon area should be avoided due to potential weakening of the tendon. Return to activity should be gradual and guided by symptom reduction and physical testing.

SHIN SPLINTS

Shin splints refers to pain in the front of the lower leg that is made worse with activity. The injury to the muscle complex in shin splints occurs where the muscle originates from along the larger lower leg bone, called the tibia. When this injury occurs in the front lower leg, as it most often does, it is called anterior tibial shin splints. This is most often an injury to the origin of the anterior tibial muscle. Pain is usually felt along the front on the lower leg. A number of mechanical imbalances can cause overuse of the anterior tibial tendon, including a tight Achilles tendon and tibial varum, also called bowleg. Hill running can also be a source of overuse. Rest from athletics, stretching of tight muscles, and anti-inflammatory therapies should be employed. Taping strategies are helpful to stabilize the muscle during activity.

The other area where muscle injury can occur in the lower leg is the origin of the posterior tibial muscle. This muscle origin is on the inside of the lower leg. Pain is usually felt just above the ankle joint. Excessive foot pronation is a common cause of this injury. Tightness of the Achilles tendon can also contribute to strain on the posterior tibial complex. Stretching exercises and anti-inflammatory therapies as well as control of abnormal foot mechanics with foot orthotics are used to treat this condition.

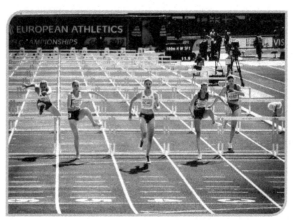

TARSAL TUNNEL SYNDROME

Tarsal tunnel syndrome is not just a sports-related condition. It can occur in anyone and is more common in the flat or excessively pronating foot. Excessive pronation increases pressure on the structures within the tarsal tunnel. The tarsal tunnel is a confined anatomic area where the tendons, blood vessels, and nerves run from the leg into the foot, behind the inside of the ankle. Chronically increased pressure in the tarsal tunnel area can lead to injury of the nerves in the tarsal tunnel, the branches of the posterior tibial nerve. This nerve supplies sensation to the bottom of the foot. Symptoms of tarsal tunnel syndrome are often felt in the bottom of the foot and can include tingling, burning, and pain. Control of abnormal pronation with custom foot orthotics is important in treating this condition. Anti-inflammatory therapies can be helpful initially for symptom improvement. Nerve decompression surgery is an option for cases resistant to conservative therapies.

EXERTIONAL COMPARTMENT SYNDROME

Compartment syndrome of the lower leg is most often related to fractures of the leg or crush injuries. Compartment syndrome refers to elevated pressure in muscle compartments that then cause nerve and blood vessel compression, leading to pain and potential tissue injury. Exertional compartment syndrome is a less severe elevation in muscle compartment pressure that occurs during exercise. Pressure increases in the confined spaces where the muscles are held due to muscle swelling during sustained exercise. This increased pressure affects the nerves that run through the leg compartments, leading to pain as sensory disturbances. Symptoms usually occur consistently after a certain amount of time after starting an activity. The nerves most commonly affected are the deep peroneal nerve and the posterior tibial nerve. Biomechanical imbalances that lead to overuse of certain muscles and subsequent muscle swelling is a common cause of exertional compartment syndrome. Reduction of activity to below the level that causes symptoms and correction of mechanical imbalances with custom foot orthotics is the usual treatment strategy.

TWELVE

Pediatric Foot and Ankle Conditions

There are a myriad of foot and ankle conditions that can affect children, from congenital deformities to neuron muscular diseases to trauma and infection. Whole books are dedicated to the subject. This chapter will describe the most common foot and ankle conditions that I see in practice in children.

INGROWN TOENAIL

The most common pediatric foot concern is also one of the most common adult foot concerns. An ingrown toenail occurs when a corner of a toenail penetrates the skin around the nail, causing pain and inflammation. Typical symptoms are redness and swelling around the nail with pain to the touch. Drainage of clear fluid from the area is common. Redness and swelling that extends beyond the nail area or pus drainage can indicate an infection. Removal of the embedded nail edge and drainage of any infection will cure it. This minor procedure can be performed in the office under local anesthetic. Very young children or those apprehensive about the local anesthetic injection may require sedation for the procedure. This condition most commonly happens during the teen years. Most children with recurrent ingrown nails tend to outgrow the problem in their late teens to early twenties. Chronic ingrown nails can also be treated with a permanent partial nail removal. This also may be performed in the office under local anesthetic.

PLANTAR WARTS

Plantar warts are warts that are located on the bottom surface of the foot. Warts are caused by a type of human papillomavirus. The virus is typically encountered in moist public areas like pool decks and showers. It gains access through the skin usually by incidental trauma such as a cut or blister. Often, the incident is not remembered. The virus causes a small mass to form from the cells of deep skin layers. This mass grows slowly and can become painful. Weight-bearing pushes the wart mass into the skin layers that have nerve endings, causing pain. The wart virus can spread on the foot and cause other lesions. They rarely spread to other areas of the body.

Because the wart mass is pushed into the skin, plantar warts are a little more challenging to treat than those on other parts of the body. There are a number of ways to treat plantar warts, from medical treatment to surgical removal.

One of the most effective treatments I have found is the topical application of the blistering agent Cantharone®. The medications in this preparation will cause a local inflammatory response in the treated area. This usually results in a blister formation of the area. Once the blister dries and the scab falls off, much of or the entire wart will be removed. One to three applications are typically needed depending on the size of the lesions. The treatment can cause mild discomfort in the treated area, which can be relieved with an ice pack application or oral analgesics.

I have found that photodynamic therapy using low-level laser energy after the blister comes off can increase the effectiveness of this treatment and reduce the chance of recurrence. In young children who may not cooperate with other treatments, an oral medication can be used. Cimetidine is a medicine developed for heartburn. It has an off-label use as an immunomodulator, meaning it enhances the body's immune response to the wart virus. This medication has been shown to be safe to use in children and adults. It is even found in OTC formulations. It does come in a liquid formulation, which is helpful for children unable to swallow tablets or capsules. I have found these techniques to be effective 90 percent of the time or more in children and adults. As with all prescription medications, consultation with a medical professional is needed prior to beginning therapy.

For resistant cases, surgical removal of the warts using laser or electrical cautery can be considered. Older children can usually tolerate a local anesthetic block of the lesions to be removed. Younger children and those with needle apprehension may require sedation prior to the local anesthetic block.

CALCANEAL APOPHYSITIS

The most common cause of heel pain in children is calcaneal apophysitis. This condition is an inflammation of the growth plate in the heel bone. It is most commonly caused by chronic, repetitive trauma like running and jumping. It can occasionally be caused by acute trauma such as landing on the heel from a high fall. Middle school–aged children are most often affected, as this is the age where the growth plate is in the process of uniting with the main heel bone. X-rays can help confirm the diagnosis and rule out other less common causes of heel pain.

The condition is self-limiting. Once the growth plate is solid bone, the symptoms will stop. That can be a few years if the condition appears early. Symptom control until the time of solidification can be achieved using a protective heel cup. This is worn in the shoe for all activities to shield the growth plate from shock. For barefoot activities like gymnastics, martial arts, and modern dance, taping the heel with a foam pad during these activities can be helpful in shielding the growth plate. Temporary reduction in activity level may be needed initially to allow the inflammation in the area to reduce. A tight Achilles tendon can contribute to stress on the growth plate. Children with a tight Achilles tendon should begin a stretching program to improve ankle mobility. Other mechanical issues such as flatfoot may need to be managed with custom foot orthotics to help reduce stress on the growth plate.

FLATFOOT

Flatfoot is a condition where the longitudinal arch of the foot is structurally flat or the arch structure of the foot collapses on weight-bearing. There is one form of flatfoot that can be present at birth. This condition is congenital pes planovalgus. In the United States, the delivering physician usually notes it and an early referral to a specialist is obtained. The hallmark appearance of this foot type is one where the top of the foot rests on the front of the leg. X-rays can confirm the diagnosis.

Treatment of congenital pes planovalgus usually includes serial casting techniques, where weekly manipulations and cast applications are performed over a period of several months to reduce the joints into a more normal alignment. Cases resistant to serial casting may require surgical intervention to allow for a functional weight-bearing foot.

People have a hereditary tendency toward flatfeet. Most children's feet look flat when they start to walk. This is due to the natural fat on the bottom of the foot. This fat gradually reduces and an arch shape can be seen usually by the age of three, which is the earliest you could assess the structure of the foot by sight. Signs of flatfoot include loss of arch height, the feet turning excessively outward when walking, the heel rolling inward when viewed from behind, and clumsy gait. Young children usually do not complain of pain from flatfeet, but they may refrain from physical activities or appear less coordinated and run slower than their peers. Older children can complain of pain in the arch or ankle areas. Pain is usually caused by strain on the soft-tissue structures that help support the foot structure.

The flatfoot can be further classified related to its rigidity. Rigid flatfoot has little to no rearfoot motion, and the arch cannot be restored by moving the joints to their normal alignment. Flexible flatfoot has normal to excessive mobility of the joints of the rearfoot. The arch can usually be restored by moving the joints into normal alignment. Some flatfeet can start out flexible and become stiffer and even rigid in later childhood. This is most often due to an abnormal bridging between two or more bones of the rearfoot, a condition called tarsal coalition.

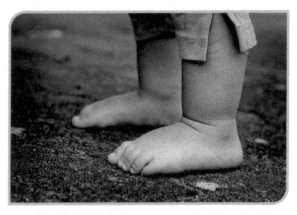

Asymptomatic flatfoot in a young child should be observed for worsening or symptom development. Supportive footwear is recommended. Foot orthotics are the first line of treatment for flatfoot. Children older than five with significant flatfoot can benefit from orthotic use regardless of their symptoms. Orthotics improve the alignment and function of the foot and allow for a more efficient gait. There is some evidence that orthotic use in children with flatfoot can allow arch structure to develop more normally as their skeletons grow. The best orthotic is custom made from a mold of the child's feet. They are usually made from firm plastics and have a deep heel cup that helps to stabilize the rearfoot. Children will usually need orthotics replaced yearly due to growth. Once growth stops in the teen years, orthotics can be used for several years with replacements based on wear of the device. Should the flatfoot not be adequately controlled with foot orthotics, bracing with an AFO may be needed.

Surgery for flatfoot is generally reserved for feet that cannot be controlled with orthotics or bracing.

There are many described surgical procedures for flatfoot. Most are quite invasive and require extended recovery periods. There is a minimally invasive procedure for flatfoot called extra-osseous talotarsal stabilization. This procedure is performed through a small incision on the outside of the foot beneath the anklebone. A small titanium implant is placed between the bones of the rearfoot to guide the joint motion to a normal alignment and degree of motion. A walking boot is used for two weeks with activity restriction for an additional two weeks. Orthotics are continued for one year, after which they may no longer be needed.

INTOE GAIT

Intoe gait is defined as walking with the toes angled toward the midline of the body. Intoeing is normal for early walkers. The position of the fetus during development in the uterus results in an internally rotated lower extremity. The lower extremities will rotate outward during normal growth and development. The average adult angle of gait is fifteen to eighteen degrees outward from the midline. Abnormal uterine position can result in abnormal amounts of internal limb or foot rotation. In these cases, normal growth and development will not result in the usual amount of external rotation. The earlier that abnormal internal positions of the lower extremities are identified, the easier it is to help "catch up" to normal development with treatment. The most common body areas for internal rotation to arise from are the forefoot, the lower leg, and the hip.

When the toes are turned inward toward the center of the body in relationship to the rearfoot, this is termed metatarsus adductus. Significant metatarsus adductus can create a C-shaped appearance to the foot when viewed from the bottom. Early treatment, while the bones of the foot are developing, can realign the growth of the bones and joints, resulting in a straighter foot.

The most effective way to achieve this is through a technique called serial casting. In this technique, well-molded plaster casts are applied to the foot and leg after the foot has been manipulated into a corrected position by the practitioner. The casts are kept on for one to two weeks and the process is repeated until the desired correction is attained. The process can take three to six months, depending on the amount of correction needed and the age when treatment starts. Serial casting is usually performed prior to the child beginning to walk. Most children can creep and crawl easily with casts on. Once the appropriate amount of correction is attained or when the child reaches walking age, the correction can be maintained with straight last shoes (a shoe that can fit either foot) for one to two years.

Untreated metatarsus adductus can result in compensatory gait disturbances and shoe wear problems in older children and adults. Custom foot orthotics can be helpful at controlling the abnormal compensatory movements. Significant metatarsus adductus that does not respond to serial casting can be addressed surgically. Prior to age three, the procedure of choice is a chondrotomy of the metatarsal bones near where they meet the mid-foot. In that area, the metatarsals are still made out of cartilage at that age to allow for growth. This type of growing cartilage heals well from surgery. The cartilage can be easily cut with hand instruments. The foot is then manipulated into the corrected position. After skin closure, a cast is applied. The cast must be worn for four to six weeks, followed by straight last shoes for one to two years. Older children and young adults require osteotomy techniques. In these techniques, the bony metatarsals are cut with a surgical saw and moved for correction. Usually, some kind of internal fixation of these surgical fractures are needed, either screws or pins. Casts are applied for four to six weeks followed by straight last shoes for one to two years.

Another common structural abnormality that contributes to intoe gait occurs within the larger of the lower leg bones, the tibia. The normal relationship of the lower tibia at the ankle and the upper tibia at the knee in adults is externally rotated from fifteen to eighteen degrees. Infants usually have a neutral to slightly internally rotated position. Natural growth and development results in the ankle end of the tibia rotating externally as we age. Internally rotated tibial positions greater than twenty degrees will not completely correct with normal growth and development. The term for this abnormal tibial rotation is internal tibial torsion.

Like metatarsus adductus, recognizing and treating this early is best. In the pre-walking child, serial casting techniques can be employed. These casts must extend above the knee for adequate corrective stabilization. These casts are harder for older children to tolerate as they restrict some mobility. The Wheaton brace is an option for children who cannot tolerate casting. This is a non-walking plastic device applied to the foot and leg that applies a corrective external rotation force. The brace is more comfortable and lighter. However, it can be removed by the curious child. A cooperative patient is necessary. Significant internal tibial torsion that does not respond to casting or bracing may require surgical management, but tibial rotation surgery should be undertaken after bone growth has ended due to the location of the growth plate at the ankle end of the tibia. The usual procedure for correcting internal tibial torsion is the supramalleolar osteotomy. In this procedure, the tibia is cut a few centimeters above the ankle joint, and the ankle end is rotated externally. Fixation is achieved with pins and a cast. External fixation is another option. Here, pins attach the bone segments to an external metal frame on the outside of the leg. The main benefit of external fixation is that it allows for immediate weight-bearing versus four to six weeks of no weight-bearing with pinning and cast.

The most common structural abnormality that contributes to intoe gait occurs at the hip joint. This is most often a soft-tissue contracture and not a bony deformity.

Tightness of the internal rotating muscles and the hip joint lining are the usual culprits. Treatment for internal femoral position involves a stretching program to relax the tight muscles and joint structures. Caregivers at home can often perform this if they are given proper instruction. Professional physical therapy evaluation and treatment can be sought as well. Activities that encourage external rotation such as bike riding, skating, and dancing can be helpful. Avoiding prolonged positions of internal rotation like sitting on the knee with the feet behind is important. Encourage kids to sit cross-legged when sitting on the floor. The bony deformity of internal femoral torsion can occasionally be present. In this condition, the top end of the thigh bone has a less than normal amount of external rotation. CT scans are usually needed to identify a bony deformity of the upper femur.

BRACHYMETATARSIA

Brachymetatarsia is a condition where one or more of the toes appear significantly shorter than the others. This is most often the result of premature closure of the growth plate in the metatarsal bone, which is the foot bone located just in front of the toe. The condition is most often noticed in late childhood to early teens as the other toes continue to grow. The condition

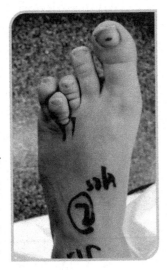

is often asymptomatic, but sometimes symptoms arise from the transfer of pressure to the neighboring metatarsals with weight-bearing. Also, the shortened toe can be pulled up toward the top of the foot, causing toe box irritation in closed shoes.

Most often, concerns with brachymetatarsia are cosmetic, and it can have an emotional toll. Conservative treatment revolves around shoe modification to accommodate the condition and insoles to balance weight-bearing areas on the bottom of the foot. Surgical intervention should be delayed until the feet stop growing. The most effective way to restore the length of an abnormally short bone is by a technique known as bone callus distraction. When a bone is fractured, or surgically cut, it begins to heal with fibrous soft tissue called soft callus. This tissue eventually mineralizes to stabilize the fracture. The mineralized callus is eventually remodeled into bone. The fibrous callus can be gradually stretched using a device called an external fixator. This device is attached to the two ends of the bone on opposite sides of the surgical fracture. It has a mechanism that can move one end of the bone away from the other. Done gradually at one millimeter per day, the soft callus can lengthen without mineralizing. Once the desired length is attained, the fixator is left in place until the callus mineralizes to stabilize the fracture. Eventually, the callus will change to bone with the result being a longer bone that is physically the same as the other bones. Depending on the length needed, the process can take three to four months before the fixator can be removed. But protected weight-bearing is necessary for an additional two months to allow the new bone to strengthen before returning to full activity.

THIRTEEN

Footwear

As a foot specialist, I am often asked for advice on appropriate footwear. Rather than provide specific brand recommendations, this chapter will focus on basic recommendations relating to features to look for when selecting footwear. As always, it is best to consult with a foot specialist or a certified fitter for specific recommendations, especially if you have foot problems or wear orthotics.

BASIC SHOE ANATOMY

Simplified shoe anatomy can be divided into the following components:

- **Outsole:** touches the road when walking
- **Midsole:** provides stability and cushioning
- **Upper:** encloses the foot

- **Closure:** keeps the shoe in place and adjusts the fit, using laces, Velcro®, straps, or buckles
- **Insole:** provides additional cushioning and/or support

Most shoes other than rubber flip-flops or certain sandals have the above components in certain proportions. All are important in the fit and function of the footwear. It goes without saying that you should select your footwear based on the activities you have planned. The following are the most frequent footwear recommendations that come up in my clinical practice.

RUNNING SHOES

Perhaps the most frequently asked footwear questions are about running shoe selection, particularly for those who run longer distances. The cumulative repetitive stresses that occur during distance running can lead to injury if the wrong footwear is used. Modern running shoe choices are numerous and seemingly daunting. A specialty running shop can be a helpful source of information if you are having difficulty finding the right shoe.

The three general types of running shoes are based on the amount of stability or cushioning that they provide. Stability shoes have firmer components, particularly in the midsole, that help restrict abnormal motion of the foot. Cushioned shoes have more shock-absorbing materials in the midsole to help people who have stiff or arthritic feet that lack natural shock-absorbing mechanisms. Neutral shoes fall somewhere in the middle, with somewhat equal distribution of stability and cushioning. The rough rule of thumb is that people with flatter feet should consider a stability shoe and people with higher-arched feet should consider a cushioned shoe. Average arch-height feet can start with neutral shoes and consider the other types based on specific mechanical issues. Certainly, if any shoe is causing or increasing symptoms, it is wise to seek the advice of your foot and ankle specialist for more specific recommendations.

Another consideration with running shoes is the so-called drop of the shoe. This is the difference in height between the heel and the forefoot. Most running shoes have a one to two degree difference between the heel and the forefoot. The zero-drop shoe has the same height between the heel and the forefoot. Negative-drop shoes have a heel that is lower than the forefoot (think the Earth Shoe from the 1970s). The higher heel of the running shoe allows for more material to absorb shock at heel strike. People who run with a forefoot or mid-foot strike pattern can consider zero-drop shoes for the weight savings of less heel material. Negative-drop shoes are not recommended for running because they can lead to overuse of the Achilles tendon. Considerations for off-road running should be looking for shoes with good tread grip, more sturdy upper materials, and water resistance.

WALKING SHOES

Walking shoes come in a variety of styles, some more sneaker-like and some more like dress shoes. For fitness walking, feel free to use any quality running shoe. My preference for walking shoes is those that are designed from a running shoe heritage. A thick, cushioned midsole in the heel is important since everyone walks heel to toe and heel-strike cushioning reduces forces that can travel up the leg. A one to two degree drop from heel to toe thickness allows for a comfortable progression to foot flat. The thinner material in the front of the foot allows for flex during toe off. The uppers of walking shoes can be made from many different materials. Choose your upper material based on factors such as anticipated weather, activity planned, and style considerations.

HIKING SHOES

Hiking can vary from a casual walk on a dirt road to technical mountain climbing. High-level technical climbing shoes should be based on the exact conditions and surfaces you plan to encounter. Someone experienced in the particular planned terrain and climb should perform recommendations and a fitting. For less demanding hiking, there are a large variety of styles to work well with different terrains and weather conditions. Obviously, cold-weather footwear should have insulation to keep the feet warm. How much insulation should depend on the air temperature and total time spent outdoors. Water resistance is also important in cold-weather footwear, as wet skin cools faster than dry skin. Snowy conditions require a higher traction outsole to prevent slipping. Warm-weather hiking demands less insulation, thus making for lighter footwear. Outsole grip can vary based on terrain and moisture levels. Though less important than in cold weather, water resistance may be needed if prolonged exposure to wet environments is planned or fungal infections of the skin or nails can result. Hiking shoes can be low top, where the upper ends below the anklebones, or high top, where the upper is above the anklebones. High-top shoes are recommended for hiking on uneven surfaces and for people with chronic ankle instability.

SANDALS

Sandals are some of the oldest forms of footwear. As with any footwear, stability and cushioning are needed to protect the feet from injury. Flat, thin, rubber flip-flops provide a bit of cushioning but nothing else. The use of these should be limited to around the pool or perhaps in a public shower to avoid contact with the floor. There are many types of sandals that have a shaped foot bed to give support to the foot structure. Sandals with straps to secure the foot to the foot bed are preferred. A strap above the ankle can provide even more stability. An outsole with a tread pattern can provide traction for different surfaces. Women's fashion sandals can be tricky. The more straps the better to provide some stability. A low heel is preferable to completely flat, as raising the heel will naturally supinate the foot and raise the arch. You should limit the amount of time and distance walked in fashion footwear.

FASHION SHOES

I am going to popularize the saying "If it weren't for pumps, there wouldn't be podiatrists." Foot specialists see many issues caused by or worsened by wearing ill-fitting fashion footwear. Men's footwear tends to be a bit more forgiving. Shaped more anatomically and generally wider, they can accommodate a greater variety of foot shapes without contributing to problems: Laced versions are preferable for their adjustability. Rubber outsoles can give better cushioning and traction than traditional leather soles. Removable insoles are helpful if a person wears custom insoles. Women's dress shoes don't seem to be the shape of any human foot. Nevertheless, they are commonly worn throughout the world. The general rule about heels is the lower and wider, the better to provide lateral stability and injury prevention. Prolonged use of heels over two inches can result in shortening of the Achilles tendon in the back of the ankle. A more rounded front will crowd the toes less, reducing pressure and friction. A deeper toe box is also helpful in this regard. Cushioning is usually minimal in women's dress shoes. Adding a cushioned insole or metatarsal pad can be helpful for this.

CHILDREN'S SHOES

Toddlers should learn to walk barefoot when possible. Obviously, footwear is often needed for foot protection. A child's first shoe should be light and flexible to allow for early walking patterns. Many toddlers start walking on their toes, so stiff soles can lead to falls. Most children learn a heel-to-toe gait by the age of four. At this stage, more supportive shoes may be needed for flexible foot types. Young athletes should wear sports-specific shoes. A low-top molded cleat can be used for most field sports. A quality sneaker can be used for most hard-surface sports. The fit should be checked regularly since children usually won't complain that their shoes are tight. The new shoe should have approximately one-quarter to one-half of an inch between the longest toe and the tip of the shoe to allow for growth. Once the toes reach the tip of the shoe, it is time to replace them.

CUSTOM FOOT ORTHOTICS AND BRACING

Many foot and ankle conditions are either caused by or can be affected by abnormal mechanics. Control of and/ or improvement of motion and alignment of the foot and ankle can help manage a range of foot and ankle conditions such as plantar fasciitis, Achilles tendonitis, posterior tibial tendonitis, Morton's neuroma, arthritis, flatfoot, cavus foot, and many others. Orthotics for the foot and ankle come in all shapes and sizes and are constructed from a variety of materials. I have used quite a variety of devices throughout twenty-five years of practice. The following will describe the most effective devices that I have found to date.

D-SOLE

This is a two-layered, self-molding insole that combines cushioning and pressure relief. It is effective for off-loading bony prominences on the bottom of the foot. These are most often used with diabetic patients as part of a foot-ulcer-prevention program when combined with extra-depth footwear. They are also helpful for off-loading an existing foot ulcer during treatment to allow the patient to bear weight. D-soles can also be used to off-load areas prone to callus formation. The bottom layer has good shock-absorbing properties. These devices are soft, so they do not provide a lot of support and mechanical control.

FOOTSTEPS™

FOOTSTEPS™ are non-custom, semirigid orthotic devices that are available only from a doctor's office. These are a three-layered device with a semirigid plastic shell, a cushioned layer, and a nylon-covering layer. These are made to fit the average arch shape. Minor adjustment in arch height can be made with heat molding. These are a good option when additional support of the arch is needed but with less need for mechanical control.

CUSTOM FOOT ORTHOTICS

These are the top-of-the-line foot appliances. They are constructed using a mold of the patient's feet to provide

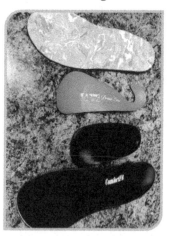

a precise fit. A variety of materials can be used and combined to achieve the desired amounts of mechanical control, cushioning, and accommodation. These can be made to fit a variety of footwear, even high-heel dress shoes, ice skates, and ski boots. These require a detailed prescription from a

trained foot specialist for the manufacturing lab to follow when making them. The prescription is determined based on clinical examination findings, anticipated activities, and proposed footwear use. This is my go-to device for the majority of foot conditions I see in clinical practice.

RICHIE BRACE®

For patients with mechanical issues that cannot be controlled with foot orthotics alone or that are arising above the ankle, an ankle-foot orthotic (AFO) can be employed. One of the best styles of AFO I have found is the Richie Brace®. This device combines a custom foot orthotic with a short, double-upright ankle 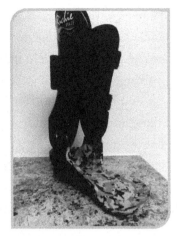 section, which looks similar to the Aircast® used for ankle sprains. The sections are joined with an ankle-joint pivot, which can provide various degrees of flexibility. A spring assist can be added to the ankle joint in cases of drop foot. Additions such as medial or lateral suspension straps can be used for certain conditions. The Richie Brace® is a custom device constructed using a mold of the foot and lower leg. It requires a prescription by a trained foot and ankle specialist.

ARIZONA AFO™

This device is a solid plastic ankle-and-foot component from the bottom of the foot to the back of the leg above the ankle with a leather internal and external liner that encases the entire ankle. This is usually closed in the front with laces. This device restricts rearfoot and ankle motion the most. These are also constructed from a mold of the foot and lower leg and require a prescription. I reserve this style of device for the most severe cases of instability or degenerative joint disease.

DROP FOOT BRACE

Patients with drop foot have a reduced ability to lift their ankle joint upward due to weakness of the anterior muscle groups. This can result in the toes catching the ground when walking, thus increasing the risk of falls. The drop foot brace is a simple solution to assist with toe clearance when walking. These are non-custom devices made from plastic or carbon fiber that combine a footplate under the foot and an ankle upright that attaches to the lower leg with straps. This device can be used with a custom foot orthotic or with the standard shoe insole over the footplate. I have also found this device helpful in any patient at risk for falls, even without drop foot. The upright grabbing the lower leg acts to provide positional feedback to the wearer, so that postural sway can be detected and corrected earlier, preventing falls.

There are a multitude of different foot and ankle appliances available to the general public. Some can be helpful and some are a waste of money. Talk to a well-trained foot and ankle specialist if you have any questions about the appropriateness of any device or to get specific recommendations.

About the Author

I think I knew at an early age that I wanted to be a doctor or dentist. I gravitated to science during grade school and high school. I also had a passion for music and sports. The medical arts seemed like a good fit for all of these passions.

I was unaware of the profession of podiatry until I had my own foot injury during high school. I was seen by a few other medical professionals with minimal improvement, when one of my coaches told me I needed to see a podiatrist. I had no idea what a podiatrist was, so I was skeptical. I was treated by Dr. Kanagis, and within a few weeks, I was better and back to competitive sports without pain. This made an impression on me.

During premedical studies in college, I thought back to my experience with Dr. Kanagis and began to look into the profession. Needless to say, I took that path and am glad I did. The practice of podiatry gives me the opportunity to help people of all ages with a wide variety of conditions using diagnostics, medicine, and surgery. There is never a dull day in my office.

I began practicing in Manhattan after my residency training. I was able to build a successful practice, eventually adding associates and partners. The long commute from Connecticut began to wear on me after twenty years, so I made the decision to leave NYC and embark on a solo career again in Danbury, Connecticut—a decidedly better commute from Ridgefield!

Since 2015, I have been steadily growing the Danbury practice, adding technology and services to better address our patients' needs. My staff and I focus not only on providing state-of-the-art care but also on providing the highest level of expertise that patients can have when visiting our medical facility.

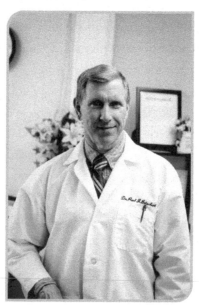